Taking Flight Through Movement

Taking Flight Through Movement

Darlene Danko Sowa, MA, CHTP

iUniverse, Inc.
New York Lincoln Shanghai

Taking Flight Through Movement

Copyright © 2007 by Darlene Danko Sowa

iUniverse books may be ordered through booksellers or by contacting:

iUniverse
2021 Pine Lake Road, Suite 100
Lincoln, NE 68512
www.iuniverse.com
1-800-Authors (1-800-288-4677)

Because of the dynamic nature of the Internet, any Web addresses or links contained in this book may have changed since publication and may no longer be valid.

ISBN: 978-0-595-47527-8 (pbk)
ISBN: 978-0-595-91796-9 (ebk)

Printed in the United States of America

You should not undertake any diet/exercise regimen recommended in this book before consulting your personal physician. Neither the author nor the publisher shall be responsible or liable for any loss or damage allegedly arising as a consequence of your use or application of any information or suggestions contained in this book.

Front Cover Design by:
Sandra Kay Bonkosky
colorsofsand48@yahoo.com

Back Cover Design by:
Cristina Pavey, Intuitive Artist
www.intuitiveartist.net

Exercise Illustrations by:
Jeremy S. Fox, Industrial Designer

This book is dedicated to my loving husband, Tom.
Thank you for always believing in me
and standing by me through my many endeavors.
Your beautiful and gentle spirit continues to enrich my life.

"Feed your body, but more importantly feed your soul. Within the realm of Mother Earth and Father Sky, the dance that leads to flight involves the conquering of fear and the willingness to join in the adventure that you are co-creating with the Divine."
—Medicine Cards, by
Jamie Sams and David Carson

Contents

Acknowledgements

The birthing of a book is by no means a solo project and it is with deep gratitude and appreciation that I acknowledge those who have contributed to making this expression of love possible.

I extend my sincere thanks and gratitude to the many friends and family members who encouraged me every step of the way. Your continued support and uplifting words gave me the courage to move forward with my dreams.

Much gratitude is sent to Mary Ellen Wojie who was the first to nudge me to move forward with my writing endeavor and whose intuitive insights and counseling kept me on track.

Special thanks go to my dear friend, Ann Burton, for believing in my vision and holding the light for this spirit-guided adventure. Your words of encouragement kept me going when the end was nowhere in sight.

A tremendous amount of gratitude is extended to all those involved with the editing of this book. Deepest thanks are sent to Don, Nancy and Kelly Danko for their insightful comments and thoughtful remarks. I also extend my heartfelt thanks to Mark Bonter for his helpful suggestions and to Terrie Voigt who so generously reviewed the manuscript twice. Terrie, your comments were instrumental in transforming a rough manuscript into a finished print-worthy book.

Finally, with a humble and grateful heart, I acknowledge my angels, my guides and all the Beings of Light who guided me along this sacred journey, always surrounding me with endless streams of love and blessings. I finally got the message.

Introduction

Did you ever think that exercise was a waste of time? This was exactly what I thought. If I had a choice between meeting with friends at a restaurant for lunch or at a park for a bike ride, the restaurant would always be my preference. Why exercise and risk the possibility of straining a muscle when you could leisurely enjoy the company of others while munching on fresh bread and spinach artichoke dip? As life unfolded, however, this non-believer of exercise found herself one day with two degrees in exercise physiology nervously standing at the starting line of a marathon and ready to embark on that monumental test of physical endurance. Exercise was no longer a dreaded and distasteful experience but had become a life-affirming practice that brought a new level of joy, enthusiasm and wonder into my life as well as the gradual liberation of my soul. The unbelievable had happened, and to the amazement of the people around me, I became an "exercise person." This book is about my journey and how I came to discover the awesome experience of exercising with spirit. It is also a guidebook for those who feel a yearning in their soul to break the bonds of limitation and explore a new world filled with pure potential and unrestricted possibilities. Moving with spirit will show you the way.

One of my favorite quotes comes from *Alice in Wonderland* and recounts an exchange between Alice and the Queen. The quote reads:

"There is no use trying," said Alice; "One can't believe impossible things." "I dare say you haven't had much practice," said the Queen. "When I was your age, I always did it for half an hour a day. Why, sometimes I've believed as many as six impossible things before breakfast."

What I like about the above quote is the sense of adventure and unlimited possibilities that it offers. To me, it states that there is so much more to life if we only open our minds and believe. And that's exactly what this book is all about—widening our perspective about exercise and our body and believing in the unbelievable.

We live in a time that is characterized by the presence of miracles. Spontaneous remissions are no longer a rare occurrence and it is getting more and more common to hear about someone who has recovered from stage four cancer or other "terminal" diseases. While it's true that medical advances do play a role in these recoveries, one might wonder: Why *do* some people recover while others succumb to their illness? Do those that recover possess a body that is exceptional or is their recovery a hint as to what the body is capable of doing? It may just be a combination of both of these.

This is also a time of astronomical physical accomplishments. Thousands of people have successfully completed the Ironman Triathlon. This is a challenge that includes a 2.4 mile swim, followed by a 112 mile bike ride, and ending with a 26.2 mile run. One of the most amazing facts about the Ironman is that most of the people who participate in this event—and go on to complete it—are not professional athletes but everyday folks like you and me. Are all these thousands of participants equipped with supernatural bodies that have special abilities? Or are they demonstrating to us what the human body is capable of doing if we give it a little care and attention and adopt an unlimited perspective.

It has been said that a diamond is a piece of coal that stuck to its job. In many ways, the body can be considered a diamond in the rough. When it is polished through exercise and healthy habits, its true essence is revealed and it begins to shine. And we begin to thrive rather than just survive. We attain the ability to conquer life's challenges, whether this takes the form of recovering from an illness, an athletic accomplishment, or finishing a report at work. But the power and the potential that is possible through exercise is not limited to the physical. In fact, in many ways, its greatest benefit rests in the emotional and spiritual realms, and this is where its impact is supreme. When we approach exercise from the spiritual perspective, we discover a new level of awareness that heightens our senses and expands our experience of life. We reconnect to our body and begin to create a life filled with joy, excitement, enthusiasm and unlimited potential.

A primary theme of this book is connection, beginning with our body, and extending that connection to encompass our entire world. Over the past few decades we have slowly learned to disconnect from our body and have instead operated largely from our head. This disconnection has been so gradual that, for the most part, many of us have been unaware of it. Increasing reliance on over-the-counter medications, overuse of television and computers, and multi-tasking have all contributed to this disconnection. As a result, we have become a society that is more productive and more efficient, yet unhappy, less joyful and emotionally empty. By connecting once again to our body through exercise, we can begin to reverse this trend and learn to create a dynamic and fulfilling relationship with ourselves and the world around us.

In some ways, this book is also about conscious creating. Through our thoughts we are constantly creating the life which unfolds before us. Every minute of the day, our thoughts are telling the universe *exactly* what we expect our life to be, and the universe obediently responds. It doesn't judge whether our thoughts are good or bad, positive or negative, it simply follows our command. And it doesn't matter if our thoughts are conscious or unconscious. Whatever thought is predominant in our minds we will see reflected in the world around us. If we are thinking that our health is largely influenced by our genes and there is only so much that we can do about it, this will become our reality. If we are always focusing on disease and physical limitation, these conditions will continue to manifest for us. If, however, we choose not to look at what has been, but instead imagine a life filled with an abundance of health and vitality, the universe will rearrange itself to fulfill our desires. The power is in our thoughts and by focusing with clarity on positive thoughts during exercise we can create by design, not by default, and transform our body into a vibrant and healthy being.

This is not to say that our genes do not have a major influence on our health. They most assuredly do! It is to suggest, however, that there is much we can do to enhance our health and wellbeing, regardless of the genes we were born with. Our genes do not seal our fate; they merely provide us with the landscape upon which we can build a solid or shaky structure. The choice is ours. If we happen to find ourselves the beneficiary of a challenging landscape, this may simply be a signal for us to give more care and attention to cultivating that landscape and taking care of our body in order to make the most of our genetic potential.

Our ability to maximize our genetic potential and lead vibrant, healthy lives has been greatly enhanced by the knowledge we have gained through science. In regards to exercise, science has proven to be invaluable. It has given us guidelines for creating a sound and effective exercise program. For example, controlled research studies have taught us that weight training helps in the prevention of osteoporosis and that cardiovascular exercise is important for both weight control and a strong, healthy heart. We have also learned through scientific research that strength training should not be done on the same muscle group two days in a row and stretching after a workout may have some benefit in relieving muscle soreness. Yet relying exclusively on the principles of science for help in designing an exercise program may overlook a very important part of our exercise experience. Science is good. Blending our scientific knowledge with the wisdom of our spirit is better. When you add spirit to a workout, exercise becomes an incredible opportunity to open your heart, connect to your inner passion and fully embrace life with a renewed sense of adventure. Spirit transforms. Throughout this book you will find countless suggestions that will help you experience first-hand the uplifting and transformative effect of exercising with spirit.

A major premise that underscores much of what is written in this book is the idea that the body and the spirit are the best of friends, and both are equally important for our overall development as a healthy and happy human being as well as for our spiritual growth. For some of us raised within the realm of traditional religion, this may be a revolutionary concept. The body has often been portrayed as the source of evil, a hindrance to our spirituality, and something that must be conquered if we are to develop a deeper awareness of our spiritual nature. Thomas Ryan offers another viewpoint.

In *Reclaiming the Body in Christian Spirituality,* Ryan shares with us that the body can, in fact, become a significant source for spiritual growth. He states that "When we use our bodies with spiritual intent, both our bodies and the occasion become sacred." Exercise, then, can be more than an activity to increase our fitness. When we approach it from a spiritual perspective, it can also become a sacred occasion that opens the way for the transformation of body, mind and spirit.

Being a trusting friend of spirit, our body is a faithful messenger, letting us know when our spirit is being stifled and in need of our attention. But more often than not, the messages from our body are either met with interference in the form of busy schedules and endless responsibilities or distorted as a result of past programming or emotional trauma. The good news is that this loss of communication between body and spirit can be changed and exercise is one powerful and effective tool that can change it. Sandra Anne Taylor shares with us in *Quantum Success* that physical exercise has the ability to "clear out old energy, and create a new, lighter and more attractive vibration (of our body)." It is this lighter vibration that allows us to recognize the spiritual in every cell of our body and thus experience a more magical and enchanting life.

It was in January of 2006 when I received a clear message from my body that something was out of alignment. It had been over five years since I followed any structured training program or competed in a marathon. Nevertheless, I felt confident that four and one-half months was more than enough time to train for a marathon. The first week of my training was invigorating and left me feeling optimistic and energized. The second week of training was another story. The workouts were exhausting and a strange pressure suddenly developed in my head. A trip to the chiropractor cleared up the mystery. My head was out of alignment with my spine and not situated properly on the axis, the bone just below the atlas at the top of the spine. To put it in more colloquial terms, my head was not on straight. My family lovingly chided me that they didn't understand why I had paid a professional to get such an obvious diagnosis!

The message my body was giving me was clear. It's great to undertake a challenging goal, but doing too much, too soon can be more damaging than uplifting to both the body and the spirit. I needed to acknowledge and accept the fact that five years without any focused training led to a measurable decrease in my fitness level. My pride would not let me concede this, so my body stepped in to deliver the message. I switched my goal to a half-marathon and enjoyed the remainder of my training as well as a successful race.

Many books have been written about how exercise, particularly yoga and the martial arts, can help a participant transcend the physical and experience a deeper spiritual awareness. But that is not what this book is all about. This book is not about rising above the body to experience the spiritual; it is about bringing the spiritual into the physical. It's about consciously connecting to the body during exercise and, through this connection, experiencing a deeper awareness of the spiritual that is always present in our physical form. When we use exercise as a means to consciously connect to our body, it becomes a powerful change agent that alters our perception and enhances every experience in our life.

But what exactly makes exercise such a powerful change agent? Clearly, thousands of people have participated in many forms of physical activity in the past and not experienced spiritual growth. And how does one approach exercise to achieve this result? The answer begins with our thoughts and conscious intentions. Throughout the pages of this book you will discover how the focus of our thoughts and intentions, along with our feelings, affect our experience with exercise and help to transform it into an event that arouses the passion in our soul and strengthens our awareness of the spiritual in our physical form. You will see that exercise from a spiritual perspective does not depend so much on what type of exercise you do, as it does on how you do the exercise.

This book is divided into two parts. Part I reviews some of the latest research and theories about brain waves, consciousness, the amazing abilities of the human body, the pliability of our DNA and the web of energy that connects, supports and influences all of existence. This is all done to give the reader a better understanding of the mechanics involved in forming and maintaining habits as well as explore the idea of what it means to be a conscious human being. Knowledge is power. Understanding more about why we act a certain way often empowers us to make different choices, choices that are more supportive of our health and happiness.

Part II of this book puts theory into practice, listing the steps involved in bringing the spiritual into an exercise program. Examples are given of how this can be done with a wide range of exercises ranging from strength training and cardiovascular workouts as well as balance, flexibility and breathing exercises. An entire chapter is devoted to developing a successful plan to assist the reader in adopting an active, revitalizing lifestyle. Finally, a list of affirmations and an example of an exercise journal page are also included in the appendix as handy support materials.

Marcel Proust once said that "The real voyage of discovery consists not in seeking new landscapes but in having new eyes." My voyage has given me a profound appreciation for the amazing resilience of both the body and the spirit, and continues to fill me with an unquenchable excitement for exploring the unlimited potential that resides within this miracle we call the human body. I invite you to join with me on this voyage and allow the gift of movement to be your ticket to a more exhilarating life filled with adventure and possibilities. Let exercise liberate your spirit, and be prepared to soar.

PART I

▼

The Theory

Someday, after mastering the winds, the waves, the tides and gravity, we shall harness for God the energies of love, and then, for a second time in the history of the world, man will have discovered fire.
—Pierre Teilhard de Chardin

CHAPTER 1

▼

LIFE AS MOVEMENT

"We all have the potential to be a full-bodied Bordeaux, but sadly most of us are satisfied being Welch's grape juice."

—Gabrielle Roth

Movement is an essential part of all life. Whether it is a tiny oxygen molecule moving through our lungs, or the earth moving around the sun, for anything in this universe to exist, it must move. Surprisingly enough, this even includes seemingly solid objects such as a wall, a table or the paper that these words are printed on. Think about it. How could wood furniture become dry and brittle or the pages of an old book turn yellow unless something moved to enable the changes to take place? If you looked at the composition of a table under a high-powered microscope, you would actually see tiny bits of energy moving at a remarkably slow speed. Sandra Taylor tells us in *Quantum Success* that "… everything (in our world) is made up of vibrating strings of energy. What was once considered to be solid matter is really composed of pulsating, energetic vibrations." So from the smallest life form to the largest, we see that movement is not only crucial for existence, it is at the heart of all that exists.

When we first came into this world, movement provided us with some of our greatest joys. It was so very much fun exploring the limits of what our body could do and we delighted in each new discovery. Our first success at rolling over not only filled us with great pleasure, it also brought smiles and cheers from those we loved. And when we took our first step, the occasion was marked with much celebration. Movement did, indeed, feel good. And so we moved on.

For some of us, somewhere between childhood and adulthood, the sense of joy and jubilation that we originally felt with movement was replaced with lack of interest and dissatisfaction. It was no longer fun to move. What initially filled us with joy and excitement now brought us displeasure and pain. Movement was reclassified as exercise, and suddenly became a chore or a necessary evil. Exactly when this transition happens is hard to pinpoint, and this is probably because it happens at different times for different people. One thing, however, is certain. Our change in attitude about movement and exercise was most likely linked to a change in the messages we received from those around us.

The Liberation of the Soul

My earliest memories of exercise were not encouraging ones, so arriving at age 30 with minimal interest or experience in movement didn't seem that unusual. This was, however, destined to be changed. On one fateful day at work two out of the three elevators were out of order, leaving walking up the eleven flights of stairs to my office a reasonable option. Or so I thought. After all, the 70-year old gentleman I worked for did it twice daily—when he came into work in the morning and when he came back from lunch in the afternoon. Reality appeared only minutes later. As I approached the third floor, extreme exhaustion set in. My heart was racing at an unbelievably fast rate and my usually controlled breathing turned into a frantic gasp for air. Walking up one more step was impossible. My body was traumatized, and I was in shock. How was a 70-year old man able to walk up those eleven flights of stairs with what looked like no effort at all? It became evident that if I wanted to experience any degree of vitality in my future, changes needed to be made.

Several weeks later I found myself excitedly standing next to other unconditioned bodies in my first-ever exercise class. The excitement lasted about 10 minutes—and was quickly followed by a monumental letdown. Did you ever begin an exercise program only to discover that it was not at all what you expected? That is exactly what happened to me. What I thought was going to be a general calisthenics class turned out to be a walking/jogging program, and I absolutely hated it. The stretches were much too difficult and the track workout was boring, and both continually left me breathless. My earlier childhood experiences with movement were confirmed—exercise was a big pain in the butt, and no fun at all.

There was no graceful way for me to quit the program. Since I was the one who originally organized the class, my pride and reputation were on the line. I resigned myself to nine more weeks of boredom and misery when something amazing happened. The stretches became much easier to do and my walking speed improved dramatically. Breathing was no longer labored. And on top of that, five pounds melted away from my figure, leaving my body looking better than it had in years. But there was something else, although I couldn't find the words to explain it. A wonderful, new surge of energy was emerging from deep within me. It was unbelievably exhilarating, more powerful than anything I had ever experienced, and it filled me with an overwhelming amount of vitality and enthusiasm. Every cell of my body began to tingle with joy and excitement. Exercise was not only enjoyable it became uplifting and invigorating as well. I didn't know it at the time, but what I had actually done was awaken my spirit. Exercise had begun to liberate my soul. Gabrielle Roth states in *Sweat Your Prayers* that "once your body surrenders to movement, your soul remembers its dance." I was remembering my dance—and a commitment I made many years ago.

About fourteen years prior, at the age of sixteen, I was shopping with my mother when we met up with one of the lady friends that mom played cards with on a monthly basis. After introducing me, the lady friend looked at mom in surprise and stated: "*I didn't know you had a daughter. I thought you only had a son!*" Those were the exact words. So what does one do at a moment like this? Do you succumb to the thoughts you've held in your mind that you really don't matter? Do you take this as proof that your life is insignificant because the people who raised you don't care enough about you to even mention that you exist? Or do you search for another answer, another voice that may only be a soft whisper but one that speaks from a point of deep knowingness. I chose the later, and what I discovered was the quiet little voice of my soul. This was a voice that said, "*You do matter; you are so much more than you realize and your life does have a purpose.*" I made an unwavering commitment that day to do whatever I could to nurture that faint voice in my soul and encourage it to grow until it became a strong and confident declaration of the truth of my being. And it was the memory of this commitment that surfaced sixteen years later during my first exercise class. Once I became conscious of this memory, I understood my joy and excitement. Exercise had begun to release the bonds of insecurity and low self-esteem and given my soul the freedom to express itself. For the first time in my life I felt liberated from external opinions and restraints. My soul was literally saying: *This is it! This will cut your spirit lose and allow you to soar!* I was ecstatic. And so I responded by moving forward with a deep desire and a passionate vision.

Immensely thrilled and overjoyed with my breathtaking discovery, I wanted to share my passion with others. It became my goal to tell others about this over-whelmingly euphoric experience that was possible through exercise and help them to realize it for themselves. This burning desire to make a difference in the lives of others and introduce them to the joy of exercise led to two degrees in exercise physiology and the co-founding of my own company. With great excite-ment and enthusiasm, I was ready to embark on my new career when life responded by presenting me with my biggest challenge. It has been said that chal-lenges are often opportunities disguised in work clothes and this was no excep-tion. Joseph Campbell tells us that "Opportunities to find deeper powers within ourselves come when life seems most challenging." I was certainly being given an opportunity although at the time it looked more like an insurmountable chal-lenge.

The Body Reveals the Secrets of the Mind

Have you ever noticed that as soon as everything begins to run smoothly in your life, and you think you have it all under control, the universe presents you with a monumental challenge. This is precisely what I was experiencing. Suddenly, whenever I began to exercise, severe wheezing and constriction developed in my throat. What an irony! My professional career as an exercise physiologist was just beginning and I couldn't even breathe without extreme effort. After discovering my life's passion and preparing for it for 6 years, it became impossible for me to do any exercise. I was devastated. The diagnosis was severe asthma, including exercise-induced asthma.

Many years later I came to understand that the onset of my breathing problem was a strong and powerful message from my body. Debbie Shapiro states in the *Body/Mind Workbook* that asthma is known as the 'silent scream,' the longing for expression coupled with the repression of feeling. The desire to expand and enter into life is followed by a contraction and an overriding fear. She also states that it may develop if a person feels smothered by too much work and responsibility. Louise Hay adds in *You Can Heal Your Life* that asthma represents "the inability to breathe for one's self." I started my pursuit of an exercise physiology degree with the belief that I really didn't have what it took to achieve that goal. The desire was strong, but my lack of confidence was equally as strong. Initial success didn't erase thoughts of hesitation and fear about moving forward. Inferiority feelings planted in youth are hard to overcome. My dream and my passion were to introduce adults to the wonderful transformative power of exercise. But thoughts of low self-esteem and unworthiness remained in my subconscious. It was as though one foot wanted to move forward, but the other foot was stuck in quicksand.

The subconscious is very powerful and often reveals itself through illness or physical discomfort in our body. The body speaks to us loud and clear, but if we aren't use to paying attention, the message flies over our head. Dr. Christine Page tells us that "the body doesn't make a mistake. It doesn't give you a pain in the neck when you need a pain in the ass." My breathing challenges were showing me that feelings long forgotten and buried in my subconscious were impacting my ability to follow through on my dreams and fully experience the beauty and joy of living life to the fullest. In other words, through the process of exercise, I realized that my spirit had been shattered. But I also realized that through exercise, that same spirit was discovering new life and learning to spread its wings.

Exercise is a rewarding and transformative experience. The resistance or lack of desire that some of us have toward exercise may have their roots in destructive feelings that were embedded in our subconscious in childhood. As will be explained in detail in the following chapter, these feelings profoundly impact our present-day attitudes, often limiting our experience of life. Through exercise, our negative feelings can be transformed into a supportive and caring mind-set that liberates our spirit and encourages it to soar. But for this change to occur, we must change our beliefs and be prepared look at exercise with excitement, enthusiasm, and a little bit of patience. Embracing exercise as a phenomenal opportunity to enrich our entire life involves gently peeling away layers and layers of mistaken beliefs that we may have carried within our subconscious for many years. These beliefs could include such thoughts as being unloved, undeserving, inadequate or not good enough. By being patient with ourselves and allowing the experience of exercise to be one of self-discovery, we permit ourselves to release these negative beliefs and replace them with an empowering, life-affirming mind-set.

A New Definition of Fitness

Working on exercise physiology degrees in your early 30s gives you a unique perspective. Most of my classmates were between 20 to 22 years old and had a background steeped in physical activity. They grew up with the *no pain, no gain* mantra, competitive sports and a "win at all costs" philosophy. Fitness meant the ability to accomplish greater and greater physical feats. My experience, on the other hand, was that there was another dimension to fitness and it was this dimension that I felt guided to explore.

There are many ways one can describe or measure fitness. Traditionally, the degree of fitness one possesses has always been depicted through the measurement of some external, objective criterion with a performance-oriented focus. Using this criterion, a person scoring high on an aerobic test is said to have a high VO2 (translated as volume of oxygen consumption) or a high level of cardiovascular fitness. Similarly, muscular fitness is often measured by the amount of relative or actual weight that a person can lift. But what about those who abuse their body by taking steroids just to receive a higher score? What about those who ingest a drug to increase their aerobic endurance? Clearly, only looking at performance results can be limiting. So, what other options exist?

Webster defines *fit* as being in "good physical condition." Granted this may be an oversimplification, but it does have a certain beauty to it. I think some of the fittest people in the world are Special Olympic athletes. Perhaps one of their legs might be shorter than their other one and they might run with a limp, but oftentimes the joy and vitality that radiates from their being is palpable. In my observations, they appear to be totally in touch with their body, at one with it, and in their own unique way, they move with a grace and fluidity that is unparalleled. Whenever I've had the opportunity to watch them compete, I've been captivated by their radiant smiles, unbounded joy and contagious laughter that flowed from them as they exercised. They experience the fullness of their physicality, and don't see their limitations but instead focus on the pure exhilaration and excitement of movement. To me, that is fitness in its purest form—using what you have to the best of your ability. In fact, I would suggest the following as one definition of fitness: *the ability to experience the full potential of our physical being and to feel joy and vitality with movement.* For some this may mean moving your index finger, for others, completing a marathon. It's all relative, and it's all about doing your best, whatever that best may be.

The West Embraces the East

When I was growing up, the common belief in Western society at the time was that strenuous recreational activity was reserved for "the athletic type," and those who enjoyed competitive sports. I wasn't athletic or competitive, so physical activity held no interest for me. Exercise was all about physical accomplishment: running faster, jumping higher, winning at tennis, swimming, football or basketball. There was also a huge emphasis placed on competition and defeating an opponent rather than striving to do one's best. I once overheard the winner of a fun run brag about beating the second place finisher and then express delight over seeing the crushing look of shock and disappointment on the face of the runner up. My heart went out to that second place finisher and I felt sad that someone would take such pleasure over another person's loss. Was this a universal attitude that permeated through all exercise and sports or was there another mind-set that honored a much broader concept of physical excellence? A look at the role of movement in Eastern culture gave me the answer.

Throughout history, Eastern culture has embraced the body/mind/spirit concept. They have always recognized that there is a spiritual energy, called *chi* or *prana,* that brings life to the body. And they have always looked upon exercise as a means of connecting to this energy, and enhancing its flow throughout the body. Whether it's t'ai chi, yoga or any of the martial arts, the focus is on both the physical and the spiritual. Gabrielle Roth tells us that the "divorce of spirit from flesh … is the loss of soul. The soul can only be present when body and spirit are one." We are much more than a physical body. When we acknowledge and allow the flow of spirit through our being we begin to connect to that part of us that gives our life meaning, that allows us to see hope amongst challenges, and that gives us joy. We begin to consciously connect to our soul.

The idea of bringing in spirit to exercise is gaining momentum in the West, and in the last few years has greatly picked up speed. Yoga and t'ai chi are becoming increasing popular, with a large variety of classes offered in most communities. Also on the rise are such mind/body/spirit exercise programs as NIA or Budokon. Creator Cameron Shayne describes budokon, which means "way of the spiritual warrior" in Japanese, as a holistic workout that combines the best of yoga and martial arts. It emphasizes the vital connection between mind, body, and spirit, and teaches you to "carry yourself more confidently, move with more agility, and rediscover a wellspring of energy."

Nia, which stands for *neuromuscular integrative action,* was started over 22 years ago by Debbie and Carlos Rosas. It is another example of what is called fusion fitness—the combining of two or more classic movement forms, such as t'ai chi and yoga. As written in *The Nia Technique,* the concept of Nia is to "use the body to heal the mind and spirit by joining muscular movement with introspection, intention, visualization, imagery, and expressiveness." It is interesting that in Swahili, Nia means "with purpose," for this accurately describes how this movement is done.

Incorporating the spiritual into a workout can actually be done with any exercise, whether its walking, biking, swing dancing or even snowboarding. To add the spiritual perspective to any workout, *what* you are doing is not as important as *how* you are doing it. By consciously connecting with your body during exercise, adopting an attitude of gratitude, adding a touch of joy, and recognizing the sacredness that defines the essence of your being, you can transform your workout into an uplifting, soul-stimulating experience. Exercise then becomes a powerful change agent that alters our perception and enhances every experience in our life.

More books are coming out that are beckoning us to approach exercise in an integrated fashion bringing in the body, mind and spirit. A good example is *Sweat Your Prayers* by Gabrielle Roth. Roth is a talented and passionate movement therapist who proposes in her book that working out "should be like having a conversation with your body and spirit; it should be personal, intimate and holy." She explains, in depth, how movement can be a catalyst for releasing stored emotions and freeing your spirit. Using movement in this manner touches the soul and encourages change in a very personal way on a deep and profound level.

The trend is apparent. More people are realizing the importance of connecting to spirit and the benefits of doing this through movement. It has been said that we are not human beings having an occasional spiritual experience so much as spiritual beings having a human experience. Spirit is our essence, and moving is our nature. By recognizing this aspect of our being and bringing it into our exercise experience, we lift our experience of exercise to another dimension and begin an amazing journey that is both liberating and rewarding. It's a journey filled with exciting discoveries, opportunistic challenges and, ideally, lots of fun. Exercising with spirit is one form of movement that will not only add years to our life, but will add life to our years.

Faith can move mountains.
Doubt can create them.
—Howard Wright

CHAPTER 2

▼

THE POWER OF
THOUGHTS AND BELIEFS

… regardless of what supplements you take and what kind of exercise you do, when all is said and done it is your attitude, your beliefs, and your daily thought patterns that have the most profound effect on your health.

—*Christiane Northrup, M.D.*

Imagine being greeted into this world with the following words: "Welcome, my precious one. We are so very blessed by your presence and honored that you have joined this family. We pledge our unwavering support to you as you embark on your sacred journey, knowing that you must follow your own path. We celebrate your uniqueness and encourage you to go out and be all that you can be. We offer you our unconditional love every step of the way. We are happy you have come to help our family grow and to teach us as we all travel this path together."

For most of us we may have been greeted initially with unconditional love, but oftentimes that quickly changed to a love with strings attached, or sometimes no love at all. As we grew from infant to toddler, many of us were fed a steady diet of "Sit still," "Stop running around," or "Stop crying or I'll give you something to cry about." The word *no* became a frequent sound to our ears while restrictions and regulations began flooding into our life. Science shares that the messages we were fed in the first six years of life, including in utero, set the stage for our life's journey. Dr. Valerie Hunt states in *Infinite Mind* that "a permanent 'body image' is completely developed sometime between the ages five and seven." These early messages then become the lens through which we view our future childhood experiences, and later our lives as adults.

Our Early Programming

One of the reasons why these messages were so firmly implanted into our psyche at such a young age has to do with our brain wave patterns. In general, the human brain operates at four different brain wave activity levels. Beta is the most active wave pattern at 15–40 Hertz (Hz) or cycles per second. This level represents a mind fully engaged in mental activity. Ideally, this is the level you are operating at as you read this book. Alpha is the next level, with a frequency of 9–14 Hz. A person resting, or watching a sunset might be operating at this level. Following alpha is theta, where the frequency is between 5–8 Hz. Theta is the level where daydreaming takes place. If you're driving and can't remember anything about the last 10 miles you covered, you were predominately in the theta state. The lowest level is delta, at .5–4 Hz and represents a stage of dreamless sleep. When someone is at either the theta or delta level, they are in an extremely suggestible state. Hypnotherapists often attempt to get their clients to reach these last two levels in order to more easily reprogram their brain and change any dysfunctional behaviors or emotions. All of us operate at all four levels simultaneously, although one level may be more predominant than the others at any given time.

In *Biology of Belief*, Bruce Lipton reports on the brain activity of children and tells us that between birth and two years of age, the human brain primarily operates at the frequency level of delta waves, the slowest brain wave activity. As a child grows from two to six years of age, more time is spent at the theta level. As stated above, these two brainwave patterns put a person in an easily programmable state. While this allows children to absorb a great deal of information about the world, it also allows them to absorb the beliefs of their parents. Whatever their parents profess, a child under six years of age will automatically embrace it as truth. Like a dry sponge that easily absorbs water, the young mind of a child soaks up the thoughts and beliefs of those around them without question. Lipton emphasizes this point when he states that "… the fundamental behaviors, beliefs and attitudes we observe in our parents become "hard-wired" as synaptic pathways in our subconscious minds. Once programmed into the subconscious mind, they control our biology for the rest of our lives … unless we can figure out a way to reprogram them." Think about the consequences of a child hearing their parents say "You are so dumb," or "You're just not as smart as your sister," or "You're always in the way." While these remarks may have been made casually, the child accepts them as "fact" and lives from this perspective.

What happens physiologically in the body and brain at this young impressionable age gives us a better understanding of the permanent effect these comments have on the way one approaches life. When thoughts and emotions are first perceived, the brain initiates an electrical impulse in one or more of its nerve cells or neurons. It is estimated that the human brain consists of a network of approximately 100 billion neurons. Each neuron can grow up to 20,000 branches or dendrites. It is these dendrites that interconnect or communicate with other neurons through the release of chemicals and in this way form thought patterns. If the pattern is repeated frequently, it becomes hardwired in the brain, and is delegated to the subconscious mind. This can work either to our advantage or our disadvantage.

Let's look at the example of a gymnast. When a gymnast first begins to work out on the balance beam, she must employ total concentration to perform the simplest movement. Her full consciousness is focused on each step. After many repetitions, the pattern becomes ingrained or hardwired, so much so that when she just begins the movement, the nerves and muscles automatically respond, and the movement now becomes automatic. It has been transferred from the conscious mind to the subconscious mind. This allows the gymnast to focus on more intricate moves and perform complex routines with such grace and ease that cause us to marvel at her ability.

If, however, a child repeatedly hears that they are slow, or clumsy, or uncoordinated, this message also becomes hardwired in the brain, but in this case a negative thought pattern is established and has a damaging effect on behavior. Chopra states in the *Book of Secrets* that there is actually a Sanskrit word for this pattern; it's called *samskara*. Samskara means "a groove in the mind that makes thoughts flow in the same direction." As Chopra explains, these samskaras are "built up from memories of the past (and) force you to react in the same limited way over and over, robbing you of free choice."

One of the remarkable characteristics of a young brain that allows it to easily form thought patterns or grooves in the mind is its high degree of plasticity or ability to adjust to its environment. This quality allows the brain to maintain neuronal connections that are reinforced by its environment or consistently used and eliminate those linkages that lack any stimulation. This is an enormous task for the developing brain and may explain why the fetal brain has more connections than an adult brain and why at the age of three the child's brain is twice as active as someone 20 years older. It remains twice as active until around the age of nine or ten when it begins to slowly decline and finally stabilizes to an adult level at around age 18.

So we see that the brain of a young child is not only very impressionable, it is also filled with an astronomical amount of thought pattern possibilities through the virtually unlimited amount of neurons and dendrites. This is the time when repeated experiences, whether they are uplifting or depressing, help fashion the thought patterns that get embedded into our subconscious. The repeated experiences and thought patterns then begin to transform our infinite mind into one filled with restrictions and limitations.

Lipton shares with us that "The biggest impediments to realizing the successes of which we dream are the limitations programmed into the subconscious." As an adult, a person may not consciously remember the comments made when they were younger, but they will continue to experience their effects. My most significant experience demonstrating the power of the subconscious mind happened when I was jogging a three-mile fun run. This was early on in my career as an exercise physiologist, and at that time my jogging pace was a breathtaking speed of around 11 minutes per mile, which was about three minutes slower than what was considered to be a respectable jogging pace. Beginning at this pace, it was easy for me to show improvement. My goal was to jog a sub-8-minute mile. After a few years, I felt that I was ready to meet that goal and had already jogged a 7:52 mile during an unofficial training run. I was confident, prepared and highly focused for this particular run. I even had a strategy. I would pace myself by secretly following my friend who I knew was a good runner. The race began and I was floating over the pavement. My stride was smooth and graceful. Every part of my body seemed to flow and work together in an effortless rhythm. I was exhilarated. I felt strong. And I was just a few feet behind my friend. We were approaching the end of the first mile, and a volunteer was calling out the split time as each runner passed. As I passed, I heard him call out "7:37; 7:38." When I heard the time, I instantaneously thought to myself, "I can't run that fast," and as soon as that thought registered, the stomach cramps began. It was as if in a split second, the entire core region of my body changed from no discomfort at all to excruciating pain. In the next second, I caught myself and thought, "Yes, I can do it; in fact I *did* do it." But it was too late. My subconscious mind was saying, "Nope, according to us, you don't believe you have the ability to run that fast effortlessly, so we'll have to do something to match what you believe." I did manage, with much struggle, to finish the race with my goal of averaging a sub-8 minute mile. I also managed to walk away with a potent lesson about the power of the subconscious mind.

The Conscious and the Subconscious Mind

The differences between the conscious and the subconscious mind are vast, and being aware of these differences can aid us in making positive behavioral changes. For the most part, the subconscious mind operates automatically, below our level of awareness. This is not only a good thing, it is absolutely necessary for survival. If we accidentally put our hand on a hot stove burner, the subconscious mind automatically initiates a reflex causing us to remove our hand. If we had to depend on our conscious mind to evaluate the situation and orchestrate a response, we might end up with second degree burns on our hand.

In *Biology of Belief,* Lipton reports that the subconscious mind processes approximately 20,000,000 environmental stimuli per second, compared to 40 stimuli interpreted by the conscious mind in the same second. If that seems hard to comprehend, think of all that our subconscious mind monitors. To begin with, it is responsible for maintaining homeostasis or a stable intracellular and extracellular environment throughout all the 50+ trillion cells in our body every single second. It controls our breathing, our heart rate, our digestion process, our filtering process, our growth process, our repair process, our immune process, and our metabolic process for starters. It does this continuously, even when we sleep. Just to perform a simple task such as reading these words literally takes hundreds of interactions which are impossible to comprehend in a flash of a second. So the fact that we do things subconsciously is a real blessing.

The reason why the subconscious mind is able to accomplish so much is because it only responds to our senses. It doesn't think…. or judge … or discriminate. It just absorbs through the senses and responds. A good example would be eating. Regardless of what kind of food, or how much of it, we put into our mouth, the subconscious mind immediately works at digesting it. It doesn't stop the digestive process if we try to drown our sorrows in a quart of rocky road ice cream. Nor does it shut down when we insist on consuming three helpings of food at Thanksgiving. When it senses food is in the mouth, the subconscious mind always responds by beginning the digestion process. It is the conscious mind that makes the decision of how much and what kind of food to eat.

The fact that the subconscious mind only responds to the world around us through the five senses is an important distinction. This means that we can't communicate with it through logic. Trying to communicate with it through logic is as effective as talking to someone in French when they only understand English. No matter how persuasive you are, or how eloquent your words, the message will not be understood. If we want to communicate with the subconscious mind, we must go through at least one of the five senses: sight, sound, smell, taste and touch.

For the subconscious mind, touch includes the kinesthetic sense. A kinesthetic sense pertains to the position, movement or tension perceived through the muscles, tendons and joints. For example, we have nerve sense organs located in our muscles that send a message to our brain when we are walking on uneven ground. The brain processes this information and sends the appropriate signals back to our muscles to contract or release, depending on whether we are walking uphill, downhill or on bumpy terrain. Thankfully, this all happens subconsciously. If it didn't, it would take intense concentration for us to even walk across a room. A champion athlete in gymnastics or figure skating would most likely have a good kinesthetic sense; in other words, the communication system between their muscles, limbs, and joints and their subconscious mind is finely tuned so that they can process thousands of messages per second and perform amazingly intricate routines. They are able to *feel* when they are off in their execution, although it may not be readily visible to the untrained eye of someone watching them.

The Importance of Thoughts and Feelings

The communication between our subconscious mind and our muscles is a two-way track. Not only do the muscles send signals to our subconscious about the position of our body, our subconscious mind sends messages through our thoughts and *feelings* to our muscles. If you are making an important presentation in front of your peers, thoughts of nervousness or apprehension may register as butterflies in your stomach. Or, if you are startled by a snake in front of your path, fearful thoughts can result in our muscles tightening.

The operative word here is feelings. Just as the muscles send messages to our subconscious about our physical orientation to our surroundings, and these messages are hardwired in the brain, the subconscious sends messages about our feelings to our muscles which are then embodied in these muscles. According to Deb Shapiro, our muscles are the physical structures that absorb and "hold" our feelings. She states in *Your Body Speaks Your Mind* that "In this way, a depressive or fearful attitude becomes built into the physical structure, which in turn maintains the mental attitude. To bring change you need to work from both sides—to release both the physical structure and the psychological patterning." So we see that our subconscious feelings are stored in our muscles, and that through exercise and the embracing of life-affirming attitudes we can change these feelings to a more supportive belief system. For this to happen it is important that we not only think positive thoughts, but actually *feel* the significance of these thoughts in our body.

It's also interesting to note that this is one of the reasons why simply *saying* affirmations rarely work. The body has to *feel* the meaning of the affirmation in order for any significant change to occur. Dr. Christine Page, author of *Frontiers of Health,* concurs with this. During a recent workshop she shared that affirmations must be *embodied* in order to be effective. They have to come from a deep knowingness; otherwise, they are only a wish.

This emphasizes the importance of our thoughts during exercise and also highlights the great opportunity we have available to us through movement. For example, if the feeling of abandonment or lack of support has been imprinted in our psyche, we can now begin to reprogram our subconscious mind by focusing on feeling supported during our exercise routine. Both focusing and feeling are key to making this change.

Let's go back to the example of the gymnast. When she's learning a new skill, she is focusing 100% of her attention on performing this skill. Every fiber of her being is directed toward this goal. If she thinks about a homework assignment, or a fight she had with her boyfriend, or doubted her ability, the goal would continue to be elusive. In order for her to succeed, 100% of her thoughts need to be focused on the outcome. She has to feel the success.

When 100% of your conscious thought is focused on accomplishing a task, the seemingly impossible can happen. A friend of mine works in the healing arts, teaches t'ai chi and has a fifth degree black belt in one of the martial arts. To earn the black belt she had to break through several slabs of concrete with her bare hand. I once asked her what allowed her to accomplish such an amazing feat. She quickly replied: "I focused on the end result. I already saw my hand on the other side of the bricks. In my mind, there was no doubt that the task had already been accomplished."

Focused attention is, indeed, powerful. In *The Heartmath Solution,* Childre and Martin emphasize this point when they say: "… the main difference between the light coming from a laser beam and that coming from a sixty-watt bulb is coherence (focus). In order to turn emotions that we barely notice into high-powered tools, we've got to learn to apply them with *focused* intention and consistency."

So if you start a walking program telling yourself "I am a vibrant human being, worthy of exceptional health," but you also have wandering thoughts about the extra pounds you are carrying, or the fact that you should be taking care of other things, the body will be getting contradictory messages and will not know how to respond. It's important that you feel the worthiness with every fiber of your being.

Sometimes our behavior can be affected by a seemingly innocuous incident, years after the incident happened. Sharon Promislow talks about this in *Making the Brain/Body Connection* when she discusses the concept of a "stuck circuit lock." She gives the example of a young boy walking down the street and encountering a snarling dog which lunges toward him. The observation of the snarling dog automatically triggers a response in his body and instantaneously neural circuits are fired, indicating an alarming situation. The exact position of the body, the muscles that were involved, the direction of the eyes and especially the emotions felt resulted in the event becoming fused into a circuit of cellular memory. Even if, in reality, the dog was no threat, each time a part of the circuit is fired up, the entire sequence could be activated resulting in a stuck behavior pattern. Years after the original event has been forgotten, a person may continue to store the cellular memory which may include a fear of walking. This could result in a reluctance to follow a walking exercise program. Consciously, they don't understand their reluctance and attribute it to lack of discipline. In reality, their body remembers that walking could be a dangerous activity. What seemed like an isolated incident that happened years ago, continues to affect their behavior.

A lot of memories are stored in our body/mind; memories that not only affect our behavior but also influence the way we perceive events. Perception, in turn, creates our reality. Dr. Valerie Hunt shares in *Infinite Mind* that "… reality is neither fact nor fiction but is the emphasis we place on various parts of our stream of consciousness." There is no objective reality. All our experiences are filtered through our emotions, leading us to our own personal perception of reality.

The Power of Perception

There is a charming, little story I once heard during a spiritual service that clearly demonstrates how perception can clearly lead us astray. The story takes place in an old graveyard that is surrounded by a high wooden fence. Growing among the graves is a large tree which showers the ground with acorns according to nature's schedule. On one particular sunny day, two little boys had climbed the wooden fence and were in the process of collecting the acorns when Johnny, another young boy, was passing by on the outskirts of the graveyard. Startled to hear voices coming from a graveyard, Johnny stopped and leaned toward the fence to see if his ears were deceiving him. What he heard startled him so much he ran as fast as he could until a few blocks later he met an old man. Johnny told the old man that he heard God and the devil dividing souls in the graveyard, and would not leave the man alone until he personally checked out the claim. Sure enough, when Johnny and the old man returned to the graveyard and listened through the fence, they heard "One for you and one for me; one for me and one for you." This certainly raised their curiosity, but it was what happened next that sent both of them running faster than the speed of light. The internal voices continued, "One for you and one for me. Well, that does it for over here; now let's get those nuts by the fence."

While the above story does give us a good laugh, it is also a great example of how our perceptions can often be very misleading. The truth is we are beautiful, radiant spirits with a loving perfection at the source of every single one of the trillions of cells in our body. If we perceive ourselves to be anything less, we are putting our belief in faulty perceptions.

When I think about perception, I'm often reminded of an experience that happened when I was around eight years old. My older brother was a cub scout and was involved in a variety of activities that led to earning merit badges. On one particular occasion, my sister and I were placed in seats in the front row in order to watch my brother and several other scouts demonstrate their "merit badge" skills. I remember feeling hurt and disappointed at the event because it seemed I was always told to sit on the sidelines, even if it was the front row. My perception was that my mother didn't care as much about me as she did for my brother.

My mother's perception of the event was entirely different. As an adult many years later, I heard her describe the same cub scout event to one of her friends. She happily recalled the event and described the love and joy she felt seeing her darling daughters sitting in the front row with neatly pressed dresses and carefully combed hair. Same incident, different perception.

Wayne Dyer advises us in *The Power of Intention* "to change the way you look at things, and the things you look at will change." Looking at it from a larger perspective, the cub scout-viewing incident was actually a demonstration of my mother's love for me. The reality of that love, however, was at that time unrealized by a little girl who had a different perception. The good news is that perception can change in an instant, resulting in an expanded vision that opens the heart and recognizes the presence of love.

When we change our perception and focus on the love that is ever-present in our lives, we also have the potential to positively affect our health by impacting our DNA. In *Walking Between the Worlds,* Gregg Braden shares that "… research indicates that specific qualities of emotion program DNA. Your state of emotion actually determines your state of physical being!" In fact, scientists have now proven that our DNA, the double helix composed of 64 possible combinations that make up our genetic code, is not fixed but is affected by our emotions. David Hawkins tells us in *Power vs Force* that emotions can be measured and classified according to their vibrations or attractor energy fields. Love, for example, is shown to have a significantly higher vibration than fear. This higher vibration is represented by a faster wave frequency and allows it to connect to more parts of our DNA, enabling the DNA to maximally support us in maintaining a healthy body. Fear, on the other hand, has a slower vibration and interfaces with our DNA to a much lesser degree. This severely limits the ability of DNA to function optimally. So we see that the vibration of love not only feels good, it also results in physical changes that enhance our well-being. The more we perceive love, the healthier we become.

Along our journey through life on this marvelous planet, we sometimes encounter experiences that can smother our spirit. We may feel rejected by friends, misunderstood by family, or criticized by someone at work. Each unpleasant experience can throw a little water on the fire in our soul, until that fire becomes a tiny flickering flame. The beauty of exercising with spirit is that it has the power to rekindle that flame and fill us with a burning desire to cut loose our spirit. We learn, through changing our perception, to freely express our magnificent spirit and let our light shine.

While we are admiring the beauty of a setting sun, there is someone else, in another part of the world, looking at that same sun and seeing it rise. Our reality is based on our perception and on the beliefs that have been programmed in our mind. The reality is that we can change the program. We can release self-criticism and replace it with self-acceptance. We can begin to recognize the perfection that is present in every cell of our body and accept the truth that we are, at this very moment, a radiant and powerful being filled with unlimited potential. As Henry Ford once said, "Whether you think you can, or you think you can't, you're right."

*"The mystery of life is not
a problem to be solved
but a reality to be experienced."*
—Aart VanDerleeuw

CHAPTER 3

▼

A UNIVERSE OF CONNECTION

"You are the light of the world."

—Matt 5:14

The body is an amazing vehicle with a complexity and ability that surpasses any man-made construction. It consists of approximately fifty trillion cells, all origi-nating from a single one-celled fertilized ovum. The process of how these cells replicate and differentiate still confounds scientists. How does a cell know if it should be a heart or a stomach or a foot and how do all of these trillions of cells know how to organize themselves in relationship to each other? Scientists have no answer to these questions.

Looking closely at some of the statistics about the body, one can appreciate the miracle of the human form. Consider that our cardiovascular system consists of 60,000 miles of blood vessels, and each blood cell covers this distance in about 60 seconds. This translates to an unbelievable speed of 1,000 miles per second. If your heart beats 70 beats per minute or 105,000 beats per day, pumping an aver-age of 5 ounces of blood per beat, it pumps more than 1800 gallons every day. And all of this takes place without the slightest bit of consciousness on our part.

Some other incredible statistics include the following:

- A single drop of blood contains more than 250 million separate blood cells.

- A piece of skin the size of a quarter contains more than 3 million cells, 12 feet of nerves, 100 sweat glands, 50 nerve endings and 3 feet of blood vessels.

- The small intestine, stretched out, is between 20–22 feet long.

- There are 45 miles of nerves in the skin.

- 300 million cells die in the body every minute.

- There are over 100 million light sensitive cells in the retina.

- Every time you step forward, you use 54 muscles.

- Adults breathe about 23,000 times a day.

- There are 10 billion interconnected nerve cells in our brain.

What is happening within the body every single second baffles the mind. It's astounding. Every second each cell in your body is creating proteins, adjusting the permeability of its membrane, processing nutrients, releasing toxins, and making hundreds of other decisions to keep a state of homeostasis both within and without the cell.

Candice Pert talks about receptor molecules, made up of proteins that are located on the surface of each cell. She states that a typical nerve cell may have millions of receptors on its surface: 50,000 of one type, 10,000 of another and 100,000 of a third. Each second all the receptors on every nerve cell are influenced by the fluid that surrounds them, and change their shape accordingly.

Every second our lungs are working hard to supply our body with oxygen, our stomach is busy digesting our last meal, our kidneys are constantly filtering waste products from the blood, our liver is simultaneously eliminating toxins, our heart is continually pumping blood, our fingernails and toenails are growing, our muscles are contracting and expanding. Every single second! And these are just a few of the thousands of activities that are happening. To read this sentence, several million neurons in your cerebral cortex had to form an instantaneous pattern that is completely original and never appeared before in your life. It would take hundreds of pages to describe what our body does every single second, yet we often fail to recognize how truly amazing this is.

Scientists are at a loss to fully explain many of the tasks that our body does on a daily basis. In *The Book of Secrets,* Deepak Chopra gives the example of the common ability of moving your big toe. Somehow, just by thinking a thought in the head, we are able, almost simultaneously to move a digit at the end of our foot. And while science can explain to us how the cortex, activated by a thought, then sends a nerve impulse down the spinal cord into the legs, feet and finally the toe, they have not been able to explain how the thought activated the brain in the first place. How did the thought first start the process? It still remains a mystery.

Chopra reminds us that the physical functioning of our body is not the only way it serves us. It also teaches us about life. He suggests that we can gain much wisdom about living a healthy and peaceful life by looking at how our cells function in relationship to each other. Our cells, for instance, obey the natural cycle of rest and activity. The heart contracts, pushing oxygen-rich blood throughout the arteries; then it relaxes, allowing the blood to again fill its chambers. If it remained in the contractile state, blood would cease to circulate throughout our body and our life would end. Our skeletal muscles gain strength during the recovery phase, not during the actual exercise session. If we overwork a muscle, we will actually break down muscle fibers rather than build them up. Rest is a requirement. To focus on working harder and not taking time to rest from the responsibilities of life only leads to a breakdown of health in some way. Our system becomes overstressed. This is true no matter who you are and what responsibilities you have. The natural rhythm of our body tells us to rest. This allows us to replenish and refresh our energy stores so that we have more to give whether it is to our family, our work environment or our community.

Our cells also teach us about equality and cooperation. The heart cell does not consider itself to be superior to a liver cell, nor does a brain cell judge itself to be more important than a stomach cell. All cells work together, in full cooperation, for the greater good of the body as a whole. They also constantly communicate with each other, through hormones and the nervous system, always keeping lines of communication open and not withdrawing from contact. They teach us about being flexible and always adapting to a changing environment. When we begin to exercise, blood is automatically diverted from our stomach to our legs and arms to accommodate the increase in activity. Our eyes continually adjust to changes in the level of lightness or darkness. The membrane of each one of our cells repeatedly changes to maintain a homeostasis in the body. Being rigid and staying the same is not a healthy option.

When you look at how the cells operate in relationship to the body as a whole, you begin to realize that these cells embody the essence of spirituality in their every action. They demonstrate for us living in balance, cooperation, flexibility, acceptance, and so much more. Observing how our body functions allows us to tap into the wisdom of the natural flow of life.

As a society, we seem to have a tendency to ignore our body in favor of following the dictates of the brain. For many of us, we think our way through life the majority of the time and approach our problems and challenges by analyzing and studying and coming to a logical conclusion. Considering what the body has to say rarely comes into the picture. Ken Wilber makes this clear in *The Simple Feeling of Being* in the following discourse.

"As it turns out, few of us have lost our minds, but most of us have long ago lost our bodies … It seems, in fact, that 'I' am almost sitting on my body as if I were a horseman riding on a horse. I beat it or praise it, I feed and clean and nurse it when necessary. I urge it on without consulting it and I hold it back against its will.

"I no longer approach the world *with* my body but *on* my body. I'm up here, it's down there, and I'm basically uneasy about just what it is that *is* down there. My consciousness is almost *exclusively* head consciousness—I *am* my head, but I *own* my body. My body is reduced from self to property."

It's important that we recognize our body for what it is—the physical manifestation of spirit; a living, breathing, dynamic organism that holds the key to our spiritual enfoldment and enjoyment of life. If we are to evolve, to increase our spiritual awareness, to grow as a species and to experience peace on earth, we must recognize and honor our body for what it is and what it can teach us. By continuing to neglect this aspect of our lives, or relegating it to a level of secondary importance, we are ignoring an important part of our development as an individual as well as the development and evolution of the human race.

Change Your body, Change the World

Written on the tomb of an Anglican Bishop in the Crypts of Westminister Abbey around 1100 A.D. were the following words:

"When I was young and free and my imagination had no limits, I dreamed of changing the world. As I grew older and wiser, I discovered the world would not change, so I shortened my sights somewhat and decided to change only my country. But it, too, seemed immovable. As I grew into my twilight years, in one last desperate attempt, I settled for changing only family, those closest to me, but alas, they would have none of it.

And now as I lie on my deathbed, I suddenly realize: *If I had only changed my self first,* then by example I would have changed my family. From their inspiration and encouragement, I would then have been able to better my country and, who knows, I may have even changed the world."

We oftentimes underestimate the transformative power that the changes we make in ourselves have on those around us. I once attended an event where a speaker talked about her experience running a marathon. Having completed a couple of marathons myself and considering the possibility of training for another one, I listened with peaked interest. She was a vibrant and vivacious young woman who bubbled over with enthusiasm and excitement about her experience. She was beginning to win me over, but it was her final statements that not only convinced me to undertake the challenge, it also put a lump in my throat. She revealed to everyone in the audience that she was in remission from stage IV leukemia and ran as a thank you to all those who helped her in her recovery. She was given a second chance at life and was determined to make every second count. She not only inspired me, but hundreds of others in the room as well, to make a commitment to strive to do our best and reach for the stars. Her willingness to make the most of her life became an example that made a difference in the lives of countless others.

There are many ways that changing the relationship we have with our body can change the world. Think about it. As we begin to take care of our body, we experience greater energy and vitality, our self-esteem increases and we become more confident, more productive. We also begin to extend more love and compassion to ourselves, to find peace amongst chaos, and to recognize more fully the beauty and splendor all around us. We become a beacon of light for others. Our triumph over inertia, depression, hopelessness, pain or suffering is not an isolated triumph. Others recognize and relate to our struggle. While their circumstances may be different, their feelings are the same. Our dedication to making a change in our life becomes a guidepost for them to do the same. What we may consider to be a personal transformation may, indeed, pave the way for global change. Sandra Anne Taylor emphasizes this in *Quantum Success* when she states that "You are—at this moment—engaged in exquisite act of personal and global creation." We are not isolated from those around us. When we positively change our thoughts and actions, we positively affect all those we connect with throughout the day. This not only includes our intimate friends, it also includes the quick encounter we have with the sales clerk at the store. Wherever we go, whatever we do, we make a difference. By being conscious of this fact we can insure that the difference we make is positive.

In *The Healer Within*, Roger Jahnke states: "We each have the opportunity to participate as an independent agent in a dramatic transformation of human culture.... For anyone, taking on these challenges seems immense, even impossible. But the first step toward improving the world is actually quite reasonable: simply, independently, and calmly improve yourself!" Change yourself, and you do change the world. Our ability to make this happen is largely rooted in our connectedness to everything in the world around us.

Every day we are finding out more and more about how we are connected and interrelated on this planet. Scientists have long postulated that an energy exists between all inhabitants on earth. This energy allows a mother to wake up in the middle of the night thinking of her son who lives across the country and is suddenly in need of her help. This energy allows monkeys on one island to simultaneously adopt the new habits performed by other monkeys on a different island. This energy allows a seemingly insignificant action in one area to effect events miles away. It has been said that when a butterfly that flaps its wings in Tokyo, it may cause a hurricane in Brazil a month later. All of these actions are the result of a powerful, all-pervasive, connecting energy.

The Interconnectedness of Everything

In *Healing and the Mind*, Bill Moyers reports on an interview with Candice Pert. During the interview, Dr. Pert offers that "…. clearly there's another form of energy that we have not yet understood … another energy that just hasn't been discovered yet …" Some scientists are defining this energy through a theory called *string theory*. The major premise of string theory is that everything in the universe is connected through waves of energy. Basically, everything is made up of molecules including the air we breathe, the chair we are sitting on and even every cell of our body. Proponents of string theory state that inside all molecules are atoms, and inside the nucleus of atoms are protons and neutrons, which can be further broken down to quarks, which are then broken down to tiny vibrating strings of energy. And these tiny vibrating strings are in essence the waves of energy that connect all life. We are all connected through the vibration of this energy. We are a unified whole, and what happens in one part of the whole affects all of existence. Because of this connection, what we say, think, and how we act has an impact on the world around us.

At the heart of string theory is the idea that everything in the world is vibration. The slower the vibration, the denser the form. Think about ice. It is made up of two molecules of hydrogen and one molecule of oxygen. These molecules are vibrating at a very slow rate, and hence, the form is relatively solid. Increase the vibration, and the ice becomes water. Increase the vibration further, and the water becomes vapor. Form and vibration are linked. The slower the vibration, the more solid the form appears. String theory proposes then that at the core of everything that exists in the universe, is not matter but a wave of energy. Dr. Valerie Hunt supports this theory in her book, *Infinite Mind.* Dr. Hunt writes that "… on the subatomic level of the particle … we cannot find the mass, and particles seem essentially empty. We find only a wave of energy without dense form."

This leads to some fascinating questions. Is this vibrational wave of energy a form of *spirit?* Are we getting to a point where science and spirituality actually blend? Are they both studying different sides of the same coin? Are we, in reality, proving that this IS a spiritual universe, and that our body has the vibration of spirit in every one of its cells? Does this give us the answer to how we are connected to all of life? I think it's interesting that more scientists are professing their belief in a "higher power." When student Phyllis Wright asked Einstein in 1936 if scientists pray, Einstein's response was "Everyone who is seriously involved in the pursuit of science becomes convinced that a spirit is manifest in the laws of the universe—a spirit vastly superior to that of man."

Einstein was not the only scientist to speak of a superior life force that permeates all of existence. Physicist Max Planck, who was honored for his research on the atom, spoke the following words when he accepted the Nobel Prize for this research: "There is no matter as such. All matter originates and exists only by virtue of a force … We must assume behind this force the existence of a conscious and intelligent mind." So after spending his entire career steeped in scientific research, Planck discloses that underlying every atom in the universe is an all-pervasive, all-powerful force.

The idea that there is a unifying, all-powerful life force that connects the entire universe is not a new theory. In her latest book, *The Field,* author and investigative reporter Lynn McTaggart chronicles the investigations of dozens of the frontier scientists who have worked in this area for many years developing hundreds of research studies that support this theory of connectedness. While these scientists have given this force a variety of different names, including zero point field, the field, or the matrix, all have agreed that it is an invisible web that connects us to everything that exists in our world.

My personal experience of the field happened on a trip to China in 1988. As part of a fitness delegation, I had an opportunity to receive instructions in t'ai chi and qi gong from the local master of the various villages and towns that we visited. One morning about twelve of us gathered in a circle for our instruction. We stood in a beginning, relaxed posture with eyes half-closed as the master circled on the outside of the circle and eventually stopped behind a member of our delegation. Even though he was behind and out of sight of the delegate, when the master moved his arms, the delegate responded in like manner. If he moved his arms back, our delegate moved back a few steps. If he moved his arms forward, our delegate stepped forward. If he moved his arms to the side, the delegate moved in the same direction. This was done in complete silence. After a few minutes of this demonstration, every member of our delegation had their eyes wide open, staring in amazement. The chosen delegate moved in perfect unison with the arms of the master even though he could not visually see in which direction the arms of the master behind him were moving. How was this possible? The answer was simple yet astounding. There was an invisible energy that connected the master and our delegate. The master was able to influence this energy that connected him to our delegate and by influencing the energy he was able to influence our delegate. For those of us who were not familiar with the existence of this energy, our morning lesson was an experience we would never forget.

Deepening the Connection through Exercise

What extraordinary times we live in. Realizing that we are connected to each other and the entire universe is an empowering insight. It confirms that we are not merely physical beings but powerful co-creators intertwined with and connected to all of creation. This connection allows us to tap into the unlimited potential of the universe, to draw from this endless pool of energy and make a difference in the world around us. And what is so exciting is that we have a tool that can help us experience and strengthen this divine connection. This tool is exercising with spirit.

When we exercise and invite spirit to be part of the process, a number of things happen to strengthen this connection to the infinite web of life. First of all, we focus more of our attention on our inner world. A well-known law of the universe states that what we focus on expands. By placing our attention during exercise on the love and beauty of our spirit that is our essence, we literally bring our spirit to life. As we bring our spirit to life, we recognize that we are a part of a greater, all-powerful force. The more we recognize the existence of this force, the more we deepen our connection to it and our ability to tap into its power.

Exercise also gives us the opportunity to release emotions and memories that may cause interference in our connection to divine source. Cell phones are great examples of interference. When talking to a friend recently who was on a cell phone, she cautioned me that we might loose our connection because she was riding in and out of the mountains. Frequently the mountains interfered with the transmission of signals and connections were often lost. In a similar manner, our negative thoughts and emotions represent interference that prevents us from feeling connected to source. It's hard to feel part of a loving universe when your thoughts are focused on anger and frustration. Exercise helps to dissipate these destructive emotions, and once we have emptied ourselves from these emotions and any illusions of unworthiness, we recognize that the only thing left is a beautiful, loving spirit. Gabriella Roth shares that "Sometimes two hours of moving were as powerful as two years on the (therapy) couch." By releasing our negative emotions, we release all interference to achieving higher states of mind and feeling connected to the field of pure potentiality.

Accessing this field has astounding ramifications. We recognize that we are a spiritual being living in a spiritual universe and have unlimited access to the creative potential of this universe. We are connected to everything that exists in the entire universe and continually act as both a receiver and transmitter of energy within this universe. We affect, and are affected by, the world around us. We, along with the universe, are both a work in progress. We can be at peace with our current state of health while striving to improve, and we learn to be at peace with the world as it learns to improve. We begin to recognize that the health of body, mind and spirit are all important for peace within ourselves and within the world.

Being at Peace in a Changing World

Being at peace and comfortable in our own body also helps us adjust to and assist with a changing physical world. And the physical world is changing. There exists a background frequency or vibration of the entire planet that some consider the earth's pulse and which is known as the Schumann Resonance. The Schumann Resonance is the term applied to extremely low frequency signals, or ELF signals, that pulsate between the earth's crust and the ionosphere, the upper most atmosphere of the earth. For years the Schumann Resonance has been vibrating at 7.8 Hertz (Hz) or cycles per second. This vibration corresponds to the same frequency our brain waves vibrate at when we are in a very relaxed state. In 1998, the Schumann Resonance increased to 8.6 Hz. In 2002, it was measured at 11 Hz, and it is expected to reach 13 Hz by the year 2012. Some feel that this increase in the vibration of the earth's pulse signifies evolution, and that our evolution is affected by, and in turn affects the evolution of the earth. Gregg Braden, author of *The Divine Matrix,* comments that "as the earth evolves, so do its inhabitants." While the significance of the change in the Schumann Resonance is only beginning to be studied, it is clear that change is taking place. Being at peace and in touch with our body helps us to be at peace and in touch with a changing earth and actively support the earth in the process of birthing a new world.

Each of us holds a power within to dramatically change our body, our life, our world. Indeed, if any change is to come about, it must begin with us, within our own hearts. We must accept fully who we are, every aspect of ourselves, before we can grow into who we were meant to be. Marianne Williamson tells us in *The Gift of Change* that "When we accept ourselves exactly as we are, and where we are, we have more energy to give to live life." Free of judgments, we then learn to live the life of our dreams. Our potential is unlimited.

One idea that helps us learn to dream again is to remember that we were made in love and this love is at the root of every one of our cells. With that information, I decided to try an experiment. I'm still in the process of this experiment, so I can't tell you the final results, but can only report on the outcome to date. It has been said that our entire body regenerates itself every seven years. Every day we are making new cells to replace those that have died. That started me thinking. If love is so powerful and even affects our genetic coding, would focusing on love allow a healthier cell to manifest? It sounded like an interesting hypothesis. So I decided that every morning I would focus on sending love to my body, thanking it for its service and instructing it to use only love in the making of new cells. I also sent the same message before I retired, imagining by body being filled with love and instructing it to use only love in all its functioning while I sleep.

To be perfectly honest, I don't remember exactly when I really began this exercise although my best estimate puts the launch date somewhere between one to three years ago. I do know that the feedback I have received to date has been extremely favorable. This feedback came from a QXTI machine that analyzes cellular health. According to the results I received from this machine, the biological age of my cells is actually 20 years younger than my chronological age. That is definitely positive feedback! And while a healthy lifestyle in general also contributed to such a good report, I know focusing on love made a significant difference.

There is much research that supports a positive outcome for my experiment. At the heart of the research is the fact that our body is composed of at least 60%

water. Some estimates go as high as 80%. This is significant because Masaru Emoto has shown through experiments and photographs published in his book, *The Hidden Messages in Water,* that the words of love and gratitude have a transformative effect on water.

Emoto began his experiments by taking samples of water from various locations, freezing the samples in individual Petri dishes, and through a meticulous process using specialized equipment, photographing the results. From the photographs he discovered that the purest water produced the most elegant crystals while some of the most contaminated water failed to form any crystals at all. Intrigued by these results, Emoto then tested the effect of words on water. To do this he wrote different words on pieces of paper and wrapped the individual pieces of paper around bottles of water. Before and after photographs were taken. In all cases the structure of the water had changed with the words *love* and *gratitude* having the most dramatic effect by forming exquisitely beautiful crystals. According to Emoto, it was the vibration of the written words that actually changed the shape of the water crystals.

Personal experience is often the best teacher. For this reason I invite you to see for yourself the effect that words can have on the internal energy pathways within your body. This can be done very easily through a process called muscle testing which was first popularized by Dr. George Goodheart, a chiropractor and founder of the International College of Applied Kinesiology. Muscle testing is based on the theory that the body will clearly reveal to an astute observer whether some object or thought will have a positive or negative effect on its functioning. One way to perform the test is to hold the piece of paper with a word written on it in your non-dominant hand while your dominant hand is stretched forward at shoulder level with palm facing down. A trained practitioner will then ask if the word on the paper you are holding will enhance or decrease your energy. If it will enhance your energy, your arm will remain strong when a slight downward pressure is applied to your wrist area. If it will deplete your energy, your arm will lower with the same slight pressure. To eliminate any interference from the mind, write several words, such as *love, fear, nature, torture, beauty, anger, peace,* on individual pieces of paper. Fold them up so that you don't know which word you are holding. If your arm goes weak when pressure is applied, put the paper in a "not good for me" pile. If your arm remains strong, put it in the "good for me" pile. After testing all the words open the pieces of paper in the two piles. You will be amazed at the accuracy of this simple test and convinced of the powerful effect of words on our internal energy pathways. To find a practitioner who is adept at applied kinesiology, you can check with holistic practitioners in your area or google *applied kinesiology practitioners.*

As stated in the first chapter, everything that exists in our world, including the paper that these words are printed on, is vibrating. We see from Emoto's experiments that this includes words as well. Whether it is the word itself or the energy or intention behind the word that resulted in the changes of the water crystals is not clear. What is clear is that what we say and what we think can positively change the structure of water, the most prevalent element in our body. What a powerful thought indeed!

Putting it all Together

When we look upon ourselves as spiritual beings having a human experience rather than human beings having an occasional spiritual experience, our whole world takes on a new meaning. We discover that unconditional love is the power that fuels every cell in our body and connects us to the entire universe. By focusing on this love, and claiming it as our true identity, we enter a new world filled with unlimited possibilities. Science is only beginning to explore this world of unlimited possibilities with frontier scientists leading the way. But we don't have to wait for science to prove what we know is stirring within our heart. We *are* more than physical beings. With an open mind and a commitment to live our truth, we can move into a new way of being. Exercising with spirit can help us move in this direction.

*"It takes courage to grow up
and become who you really are."*
—e. e. cummings

CHAPTER 4

▼

THE WHIRLING ENERGIES OF LIFE

"What the caterpillar calls the end of the world, the master calls a butterfly."

—Richard Bach

In addition to our physical body, we each have a higher vibrational subtle energy body which surrounds and permeates our physical form. It is this energy body that actually acts as a template for the development of our physical form. Similar to the way the construction of an office building follows the details of a blueprint our body takes shape as dictated by this template of energy. Anything that we experience in our physical body we first experience in our energy body. It is also through this subtle body, this energy field, that we are connected to and receive "life force" or what the Eastern culture calls *prana* or *chi*. Located within the subtle body are whirling vortices called chakras, and it is the chakras that act as transmitters of energy from divine source.

Chakra is a Sanskrit term which means "wheel" or "disk." In *Chakra Balancing*, Anodea Judith describes the chakras as "centers of organization for the reception, assimilation and expression of life force energy." Inherent in this description is the recognition that at its most basic level, the body is pure energy, and receives energy through the chakras from a higher source. Dr. Richard Gerber, a physician who has researched alternative therapies for many years, concurs in *Vibrational Medicine* stating that the chakras are "somehow involved in taking in higher energies and transmuting them to a utilizable form within the human structure." There are seven major chakras in the body that represent the main areas where this spiritual energy interfaces with the physical.

The seven major chakras are located along the spine, and are sometimes pictured as a funnel with the tip of the funnel resting on or above the spine and the wider mouth of the funnel 4 to 6 inches above the body. Some feel it is the spinning motion of these chakras that allows the life force to enter our physical body. The healthier we are, the more vibrant and steady is their spin. Just like our body stores our emotions and memories, it has been said that within each chakra our own personal stories, including our triumphs and disappointments, our successes and failures, are also stored. Through movement we have an opportunity to release self-limiting memories and spin new stories.

While most people cannot physically see the chakras and these "wheels of energy" won't show up on any x-ray or MRI, they do have a correlation to a physical component of the body. This became apparent one day to Dr. Candice Pert, author of Molecules of Emotions. While Dr. Pert was working at the National Institutes of Health (NIH), she had a chart posted in her office of the human body which displayed seven central nerve ganglia, or bundles of nerves, branching out from the spinal column. She was studying opiate receptors located on the membranes of nerve cells and the chart pinpointed the seven areas in the body where a preponderance of nerve fibers existed. She knew nothing of the chakra system. An Eastern Indian visitor walked into her office one day and was surprised to see the chart of the human body highlighting, in his mind, the seven chakras. Indeed, when the young visitor pulled out his chart of the chakra system, they both discovered that they were talking about the same areas of the body. The charts matched perfectly.

Although there are hundreds of chakras throughout the body, in this book we will focus on the seven major ones that are located in the center of the body, running up the spine from the coccyx to the top of the head. These seven major chakras are: the base or root chakra, the sacral chakra, the solar plexus chakra, the heart chakra, the throat chakra, the third eye chakra and the crown chakra. Each of these chakras not only governs a particular area in the body, it also represents specific emotions and qualities. For example, the solar plexus chakra, located in the area around the navel, can enhance self-confidence and assertiveness while a healthy throat chakra can encourage clear and honest communication. Knowing what chakra influences the muscle you are working on, and what qualities that chakra represents, will enable you to bring more life and vitality into your body and add another aspect to your workout. You will begin to understand that the spiritual and physical are intricately intertwined into one beautiful expression of life. Following is a brief summary of each of the seven major chakras.

The Root Chakra (Sanskrit name: muladhara)

Key words: safety, survival, grounding
Element: earth
Color: red
Associated body parts: legs, bones

Located at the base of the spine, the root chakra is associated with our most basic instinct—survival. It reflects our ability to be grounded and feel safe both in our body and in the world. Many of us have a hard time connecting with our bodies so working with this chakra is very important if we want to recognize the gift of our physical form. This was brought home to me while working as an exercise physiologist at a multi-disciplinary weight control clinic. One day two different clients did not want to feel their pulse, even though it was explained to them that this would be a good way to check their heart rate. They were frightened at the prospect of getting in touch with their body in this simple way. Confused, I asked the resident psychologist to enlighten me, without revealing any confidential information about the clients. Her comment was an eye-opener. She said that oftentimes when someone is physically or emotionally abused, they will totally disconnect from their body in order to cope with the trauma. While many of us may not have a history of extreme abuse, we may have a number of traumatic memories which left us feeling uncomfortable about our bodies.

Anodea Judith tells us in *Chakra Balancing* that "To deny your body is to be a 'no-body'. Honoring your body as the sacred temple for the divine within you is the primary task of the first (root) chakra. If your vehicle is in order, the journey is more enjoyable."

So this chakra is about feeling comfortable with our existence in our body, on the earth plane, and recognizing that this existence is the physical manifestation of a divine spirit.

Any exercise that works to strengthen or stretch the muscles of the back or the legs, particularly the quadriceps, the hamstrings, and the calf muscles, will help to deal with issues of this chakra. Some of these issues include obesity, anorexia, workaholism, excessive spending and resistance to change or structure. Characteristics of a balanced root chakra include groundedness, being comfortable in your body, a healthy sense of safety and security, and prosperity.

Strengthening our legs are important first steps in feeling comfortable in our body and claiming our identity. I find it very interesting that at this time when more women are focusing on their own empowerment, there are also more women focusing on their physical strength. The two go hand in hand. As Karen

Andes points out in *A Woman's Book of Strength*, "This journey into strength is not just about sculpting the body but how we can use the "pathway" of our bodies as a way to mine the strength in ourselves. For when external and internal strength are blended and balanced, the wires connect, the whole person wakes up and that union of flesh and spirit is magnificent, radiant, a course to rejoice." What inspiring words!

The Sacral Chakra (Sanskrit name: svadhisthana)

Key words: movement and fluidity
Element: water
Color: orange
Associated body parts: lower back, bodily fluids, sex organs

The sacral chakra is located in the lower abdomen. While the root chakra confirms our presence in the world, the sacral chakra begins to define that presence through the act of moving. Movement is not only a requirement for life to exist, it is also essential in order for us to experience and evolve our spiritual selves. The way we physically move is closely related to the way we move through life in general.

In animal lore, the grouse represents the sacred power of movement. Many Plains Indians perform the Grouse Dance to honor these birds and experience a heightened consciousness. Jamie Sams and David Carson share with us in *Medicine Cards* that grouse medicine is an invitation to dance and contemplate how our dance with life harmonizes with the rhythms or dance of mother nature.

Exercise in general is a sacral chakra activity since all exercise involves movement. Cardiovascular exercise in particular helps to address the issues of this chakra. These issues include excessive mood swings, poor boundaries, rigidity in body and behavior and boredom. Characteristics of a balanced sacral chakra include graceful movements, confidence, healthy boundaries, warmth and ability to embrace change.

The Solar Plexus Chakra (Sanskrit name: manipura)

Key words: self-esteem, assertiveness, discipline, vitality
Element: fire
Color: yellow
Associated body parts: abdomen, lower and middle back, digestive system, liver, spleen, gallbladder and adrenal glands

The solar plexus chakra is located in the area of the navel and is associated with our personal identity and self-esteem. This chakra is also known as the "power center" and is the place where you build your strength on all levels and develop your will. It is the chakra of the mind, ruling rational thought, and also the chakra of the digestive system and metabolism. Because this chakra rules the mind and is the center of intellect and decision-making, making our own choices as opposed to having them made for us is important for the healthy development of this chakra and for the development of our own individuality.

The abdominal area includes the digestive system and middle and lower back as well as the abdominal muscles. This is the area where we process our reality, acting on what we have digested in food and thought. Oftentimes, our inability to digest what we see and feel around us leads to such physical problems as gallstones, arthritis, ulcers and digestive problems.

Any exercise that works the abdominal muscles helps to deal with issues of this chakra. These issues include poor self-image, arrogance, indecisiveness, powerlessness, lack of energy, and poor digestion. Characteristics of a balanced solar plexus chakra include energetic, confident, warm, self-disciplined, responsible, and spontaneous.

The Heart Chakra (Sanskrit name: anahata)

Key words: love, compassion, peace, contentment, acceptance
Element: air
Color: emerald green
Associated body parts: heart, lungs, chest, shoulders, arms, upper back

The heart chakra is located in the center of the chest and is also the center of the seven major chakras in the body. The three chakras below this energy center represent the personal and the physical while the three above it embody the spiritual and the universal. So this chakra has been known as the balance center between the physical and the ethereal, the fundamental link between the physical and the transcendental, the body and the spirit.

The major emotions associated with this chakra are love and compassion and this energy center concerns our ability to give and receive in all areas of our life. This is where our innermost feelings of the heart are outwardly expressed, traveling first through the shoulders and then down the arms and out the hands.

Exercises that help to deal with issues of this chakra include all cardiovascular exercises as well as exercises involving the shoulders, chest, arms and upper back. These issues include jealousy, codependency, loneliness, critical behavior, unforgiveness and fear of intimacy. Characteristics of a balanced heart chakra include love, compassion, peacefulness and contentment.

The Throat Chakra (Sanskrit name: vissudha)

Key words: expressing, clear communication, creativity
Element: ether
Color: turquoise or blue
Associated body parts: throat, neck, ears, jaw, mouth, teeth, thyroid gland

The throat chakra is located in the hollow area of the throat and represents our ability to clearly and honestly communicate and express our thoughts and ideas. It also represents our ability to speak our truth with conviction and listen with a compassionate heart. Being the first of the higher or universal chakras, this area is responsible for the development of our unique inner voice and communication on a spiritual level.

The word vocation comes from the Latin word *voca* which means voice or calling. When the throat chakra is balanced people often suddenly discover a fresh outlook on what they want to do in their own life. They respond to an inner voice which is clearly calling them to fully express who they are in their own unique way.

The muscles associated with this chakra include the neck muscles as well as the vocal cords. Singing and toning are excellent ways to deal with the issues of this chakra. These issues include fear of speaking, tone deafness, stuttering, talking too much and excessive shyness. Characteristics of a balanced throat chakra include good communication with self and others, a resonant full voice, good listening skills and creativity.

The Third Eye Chakra (Sanskrit name: ajna)

Key words: wisdom, inner sight
Element: light
Color: indigo
Associated body parts: face, eyes, brain, pituitary and pineal glands, lymphatic and endocrine systems

The third eye chakra is located between and above the eyes and represents our ability to see both internally and externally, to develop a clear, personal vision and to trust our intuitive wisdom.

It has been said that the eyes are the windows to the soul, and, indeed, they express every emotion that we experience. They are also the means through which we see the reality of the world around us. When this chakra is balanced, we not only see clearly what surrounds us but we also look beyond ordinary vision into the subtler realms of energy and spirit. This is the area of intuition, dreams and visions.

The third eye chakra is also associated with the brain. When this area is balanced it can lead to extraordinary clarity of thought and the combining of logical reasoning with intuition and inspiration. We are able to see clearly in the deepest sense.

The eyes and the brain are two of the body parts that help to deal with issues of this chakra. These issues include lack of imagination, difficulty concentrating, denial, intellectual stagnation or decline, and confusion. Characteristics of a balanced third eye chakra include strong intuition, good memory, penetrating insight and clear vision.

The Crown Chakra (Sanskrit name: sahasrara)

Key words: realization, infinity, peace and fulfillment
Element: energy
Color: white or violet
Associated body parts: center of the head, brain, fontanel

The crown chakra is located at the top of the head and is known as the *thousand-petaled lotus* which is the symbol of purity and spirituality. This chakra represents our ability to achieve deep understanding, inner wisdom and a connection to the highest state of enlightenment and spiritual growth on the earth plane. It represents our willingness to surrender to divine will and experience a oneness with the universe.

In newborn babies the soft spot on top of the head, called the fontanel, is the place where the bones of the skull have not yet fused together. This allows light from divine spirit to enter the body. Through visualization, we can reopen this spot on our head as a symbol of our opening up to divine spirit and inspiration. This symbolic gesture allows us to receive guidance from spirit, often clarifying our true purpose in life and experience the wonder and rapture of existence.

Issues related to this chakra include confusion, living "in your head", disconnection from spirit, excessive attachments, a closed mind and rigid beliefs. Characteristics of a balanced crown chakra include wisdom, open-mindedness, and a deep spiritual connection.

In some ways our energy body is much more complex and intricate than our physical body. Just as we are continually discovering something new about our physical form, we are also constantly expanding our knowledge of the energy field that underlies that form. Our knowledge about this energy around and within our body is in its infancy and in truth is changing just like our physical body is changing. For this reason, I urge you to use this information as a guide to enhancing your workouts and always follow what resonates as truth in your heart. Some say the lower back is associated with the sacral chakra, and some say it is associated with the solar plexus chakra. Both are probably right. Rather than being absorbed with seemingly conflicting bits of information, listen to what rings true for you. In the final analysis, you are the expert on the workings of your body.

For Further Reading

There are many excellent books that explore the chakra system as well as books that approach working with the body from a holistic perspective. Below are some of my favorites. They will all add to your understanding and enjoyment of the miracle of the human body.

My favorite strength book is *A Woman's Book of Strength* by Karen Andes. As the subtitle states, this book is "an empowering guide to total mind/body fitness." Andes not only covers the mechanics of a resistance workout in exquisite detail, she frames the exercises in the context of a total life experience, even including a meditation at the end of the book for "the fully realized woman." This book takes strength training to another dimension.

One of the easiest to use tools that I have discovered on the subject of exercise and the chakra system is the *Chakra Deck* by Olivia Miller. This convenient deck of 50 cards is a great tutorial for the chakra system, giving detailed descriptions, breathing and movement exercises as well as meditations for each chakra. It's both handy and informative.

For more in-depth information on the chakra system, Anodea Judith's *Chakra Balancing Kit* is invaluable. The workbook for this kit is filled with in-depth information on each chakra, including sections explaining excessive and deficient characteristics of each energy center, the psychological issues involved, and pointers on how to deepen your connection with these "wheels of light."

Another excellent resource is *The Chakra Energy Plan* by Anna Selby. This book contains detailed descriptions of the seven main chakras as well as yoga and t'ai chi exercises that work to balance and revitalize these centers.

A standard reference in the Healing Touch community is Debbie Shapiro's book, *Body/Mind Workbook*. This book is one of the *bibles* used by energy workers. It describes in great detail how the mind and the body work together and includes detailed descriptions of the significance of illness and disease on the human form. This is a great reference book to keep on hand. Shapiro's latest book, *Your Body Speaks Your Mind,* takes the body/mind relationship one step further, providing poignant questions designed to assist the reader in deepening their own spiritual awareness.

PART II

▼

The Practice

"How do geese know when to fly to the sun? Who tells them the seasons? How do we, humans know when it is time to move on? As with the migrant birds, so surely with us, there is a voice within if only we would listen to it, that tells us certainly when to go forth into the unknown."
—Elizabeth Kubler Ross

CHAPTER 5

▼

THE SPIRITUAL PERSPECTIVE

"A bird doesn't sing because it has an answer, it sings because it has a song."

—Maya Angelou

When I worked actively in the wellness field delivering corporate and community wellness programs, there was a diagram that I often referred to called the Wellness Continuum. This diagram consisted of a single horizontal line, with the center point of the line representing absence of disease, the farthest left point indicating death and the farthest right point indicating high level wellness. The theory was that the farther right you were along the continuum, the healthier you were. Allopathic medicine could help you get to the center, but you had to make some lifestyle changes if you wanted to continue moving right. In other words, if you had a severe heart attack as a result of blocked coronary arteries, a surgeon could mend the arteries by performing by-pass surgery. But if you wanted to strengthen the heart, you would have to begin a cardiovascular exercise program. The same could be said of your muscles and bones. A physician could help set a broken bone, but for stronger bones, diet and exercise are important. In other words, in order to achieve high level wellness we need to be proactive.

Death	Absence of Disease	High Level Wellness

We can take this same diagram and modify it to signify our spiritual awareness as shown below. The farthest point on the left, *devoid of spirit*, now represents someone who mechanically goes through life feeling alone and disconnected to any spiritual source. Their life lacks meaning and they often feel powerless. In contrast, the point on the extreme right, *spiritual enlightenment*, represents those individuals who feel a deep connection to a higher power. These are individuals who radiate a warmth and compassion to those around them and bring beauty and joy to every encounter. Their mere presence exudes a pure and genuine love that transforms all that surrounds them. The Dalai Lama is a good example of this state of existence.

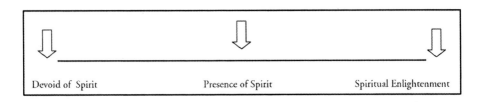

Now consider this. The same positive lifestyle habits can help us move farther to the right on both diagrams. For example, consistently following a walking program will not only improve the function of your heart muscle, it can also increase the feeling of peace within the heart. Meditation not only helps us connect to the divine source within us, it also reduces the level of stress chemicals circulating in our body. Eating a healthy diet helps us to feel lighter both physically and spiritually. The fact that the same activity that benefits the physical also benefits the spiritual demonstrates that there is a definite connection between our body and our spirit.

This connection is not a new concept but one that has been embraced by various cultures throughout history including Native Americans. Many of these native cultures look upon sickness and physical ailments as a spiritual crisis and address both the body and the spirit in treating diseases or physical challenges. More recently a number of authors have written extensively on this connection with Debbie Shapiro and Louise Hay being two of the most well-known in this area. Using the same example of a heart attack, Shapiro states that this health crisis usually occurs "at a time of financial pressure and competition, combined with a growing alienation from family and loved ones." She continues that this problem indicates a need to slow down and reevaluate what's really important as well as learning to love oneself more and share that love with others. Shapiro points out that heart attacks have increased in the West as we have become obsessed with achievement and material gain. Louise Hay adds a slightly different perspective suggesting that a heart attack symbolizes squeezing all the joy out of the heart in favor of money or position.

But what if you haven't had a heart attack or any heart problems? Can strengthening the heart, and moving farther to the right on the graph, also enhance our spiritual growth? Will increasing the strength of our muscles also increase the strength of our spirit? Does actively working to increase our health also assist us in raising our vibration and experiencing greater spiritual awareness? No matter where you are on the graph, the answer to these questions is a definite *yes*.

We hear much more about the physical and emotional benefits of exercise than we do about any spiritual gains. A regular exercise program can increase your cardiovascular health, strengthen your muscles, protect you against osteoporosis, help reduce blood pressure and control cholesterol, improve balance and flexibility and reduce stress. But it can also ignite a passion within you, give you a profound feeling of peace, stimulate an unwavering hope for the future, increase your capacity to love, and provide you with a greater sense of courage, strength and unbounded joy. These later benefits are all the result of bringing spirit into your exercise program. In some ways, not including the spiritual as part of your exercise is like riding around the countryside on a wonderful, warm summer day in a convertible with the top up. The ride may be enjoyable, but you can experience so much more by taking the top down, gazing up at a gorgeous blue sky, feeling a refreshing breeze kiss your cheeks, and allowing your senses to more fully connect to the beauty of nature.

Exercise can indeed be a catalyst to our physical, emotional and spiritual growth. By following four simple steps we can maximize the benefits we receive from our movement program and experience a new dimension to every workout. These steps will guide you on a path that embraces spirit every step of the way.

The Four Steps to Exercising with Spirit

Embracing the spiritual aspect of exercise has more to do with *how* you do an exercise than *what* specific exercise you do. While exercises like yoga and t'ai chi seem naturally geared to blend the spiritual with the physical, any exercise can be done incorporating both of these areas. There are four simple ways to make this happen and transform your workout into a spiritual experience. To add the spiritual, exercise must be done in a manner that recognizes the body as sacred; it must be done with an attitude of gratitude; it must be pleasurable and include joy; and, it must embrace the present moment.

1. Recognize the Body as Sacred

For some of us, it's a lot easier to see the presence of the divine in everything else than it is to witness it in our body. We recognize the existence of spirit in the splendor of a sunset, the beauty of a budding flower, or the playful movements of children in the park. We can even see it in a blade of grass or leaves on a tree. But for some reason, it's hard for us to imagine this same divine spirit in our fingernails, our thighs, our arms, or our hair. The truth is, every single cell in our body is made out of divine love and, therefore, has pure love as its essence. When we are aware of the divinity at our source, not only intellectually but emotionally as well, we develop a reverence for our body that leads us to treat it with tender loving care (TLC) in all that we do—including exercise.

In practical terms, treating the body with TLC begins with nurturing it with proper food and clothing. Imagine that you own a beautiful, vibrant champion race horse. One of your greatest pleasures is seeing its sleek body effortlessly run on the track, with the grace and ease of an eagle riding the currents of the wind. To keep such an exquisite horse performing well, you would make sure it was properly nourished and regularly groomed. The horseshoes would be replaced at the slightest hint of wear and tear. Well, your body is more valuable than any race horse that ever existed. So take special steps to make sure you provide your body with high quality food and water, along with the proper shoes and clothing before, during and after you exercise.

Recognizing the body as sacred and treating it with TLC also means being kind and gentle with your body during exercise, and not judging what you can do in relationship to others. This can sometimes be a challenge when exercising in a group. In a group setting we may be tempted to over-extend ourselves in order to keep up with others. It's important to feel happy and comfortable with what you can do at the moment, regardless of what anyone else can do. Physical improvement is an important part of exercise, but overdoing it is not a recommended means to accomplish this. At one time or another, we have all experienced the repercussions of stretching too far, running too fast or lifting too much. And while we may have learned our lesson in the past, sometimes our memory fades as time passes on. Always remember the sacredness of the body as you go through your workouts. If you find that you are comparing your actions and performance to others, this may be a signal that you are not listening to and honoring your own body. As you strive to improve, be gentle and kind to your body and it will respond with appreciation.

2. Adopt an Attitude of Gratitude

The attitude of gratitude is probably one of the easiest principles to incorporate into your exercise session, and one whose benefits are well documented. Masaru Emoto shares with us in *The Hidden Messages of Water* that expressing thoughts of gratitude to water, whether in a bottle or in a lake, actually change the crystal-line form of the water to its most perfect form, a beautiful hexagonal shape. In a similar fashion, thoughts of love and gratitude can actually change the cells in our body. Gregg Braden states in *The Divine Matrix* that "Research has shown beyond any reasonable doubt that human emotion has a direct influence on the way our cells function in our body." So sending thoughts of appreciation and gratitude to different parts of our body has the potential to greatly improve its function.

My experience with expressing gratitude during exercise has always brought positive results, especially on days when I really didn't think I had the energy to work out. Sending thanks to my legs for allowing me to walk forward in my life, to my heart for pumping oxygen-rich blood to each and every cell, to my lungs for supplying my body with the breath of life, to my liver and kidneys, and eyes and ears is a great energy boost and invariably has the most wonderful uplifting effect. It's almost as if thoughts of gratitude are waking up the individual body parts and bringing them new life. At the least, this is a great way to bring a fresh perspective to your workout.

3. Add Pleasure and Joy

If you decided to do only one thing to add the spiritual dimension to your work-out, adding joy and pleasure would probably be a good choice. It's hard to under-estimate the power of joy because this is what brings your spirit to life and allows it to dance with delight. It can transform your workout into a magnificent experi-ence.

When I recently asked a number of people what exercise meant to them throughout their life, joy and pleasure were frequently mentioned. One woman responded that when she participated in activities that she enjoyed, she really didn't consider it exercise, but rather a time to fully engage in life and feel the joy of being alive. If the activity was fun and brought her enjoyment, the chances are that she would do it more consistently. In fact, she would make sure that other events in her life did not intrude on her joyful experience.

Joy is all about unleashing your spirit and letting it soar. It's about doing something that gives you pleasure and feeds that spirit. Exercise doesn't have to mean walking, swimming or biking workout sessions. It can also mean ballroom dancing, tennis lessons, playing Frisbee, or even joining a hockey league. A friend of mine who is over 50 years old told me recently that she just began playing hockey on a woman's league, and absolutely loves it! With enough padding to qualify as a Pillsbury doughboy look-a-like, she shared that it was so much fun because the enormous amount of cushion that surrounded her body allowed her to bump and fall and not feel even a hint of pain. She felt like a kid again. To her, hockey was not just exercise, it was play. Find the activity that feels like play to you and you have found your key to joy.

Play is, in fact, a very important part of life. Dr. Thomas Armstrong proposes in *The Human Odyssey* that "Play is the critical factor not only in the development of individuals but also in the creation of civilizations." It is a playful attitude that allows us to reach the height of our creative potential and bring the magic back in our lives. The nature of play itself entices us to take things lightly and become more relaxed and uninhibited. It also unleashes a creative process that leaves the door open to new and exciting possibilities. This is because play has no rules, at least none that are written in stone. It simply beckons you to have fun.

Even if the only form of activity that is conveniently available to you is walking, you are virtually unlimited in ways to add joy to your workout. Thanks to such inventions as the iPod and MP3 players, you can make your exercise sessions more enjoyable by listening to an infinite selection of music, books, inspiring lectures and entertainment. Another friend of mine reported that she walked an extra twenty minutes on the treadmill one day because she was listening to a mystery novel and wanted to find out what would happen next. She promised herself that she would only listen to the novel while exercising, so when the suspense escalated, extending her walking was the only way she had of discovering the outcome of the story.

You can also add joy by wearing something special that makes you smile. One of my favorite workout clothes is a t-shirt which has a picture of a queen on the front with the caption, "It's good to be queen" underneath it. This is my "designated exercise t-shirt" that is only worn during my workouts. It was a gift to me and makes me feel good whenever I wear it. Find what makes you feel special and reserve it for your exercise sessions. It doesn't even have to be a piece of clothing, but could also be a pendant or a crystal that you put in your pocket. The only requirement is that it reminds you of how precious you are and brings you joy.

4. Embrace the Moment

The fourth step to exercising from the spiritual perspective is to be totally present, and fully aware of how you feel both physically and emotionally as you exercise. Pay attention to what is happening in the present moment. When you are fully present during your workout, you experience an intensely alive state where every action becomes an expression of high-spirited energy. You are aware of the rhythm of your breathing, of the air flowing in and out of your body. You feel your muscles guide your body through its movements. You notice when any constriction or tightness occurs and gently make adjustments so that all resistance dissolves. You learn how to listen to the body and respond with love. This is when real transformation, of you and your workout, takes place. As Eckert Tolle shares with us in *The Power of Now,* "As soon as you honor the present moment, all unhappiness and struggle dissolve, and life begins to flow with joy and ease. When you act out of present-moment awareness, whatever you do becomes imbued with a sense of quality, care, and love—even the most simple action." Keeping your attention clearly focused on the present when you are exercising allows you to embrace the infinite creative potential of the present moment and transforms your workout into a joyous celebration of life.

In summary, any workout can be transformed into a spiritual experience. For this to happen, you must treat the body as sacred, adopt an attitude of gratitude, always move with joy, and embrace the present moment. By integrating these four principles into your workout, you will discover a new dimension to your exercise that will put a smile on your face, joy in your heart and a spring in your step. You will discover your spirit.

"Now here is my secret, very simply: you can only see things clearly with your heart. What is essential is invisible to the eye."
—The Little Prince

CHAPTER 6

▼

EXERCISING WITH SPIRIT

"Living in strength gives us no need to wear armour, but the courage to reveal ourselves as we are."

—Karen Andes

We've covered the theory. Now we're ready to put it into practice. The four steps to exercising with spirit can basically be boiled down to three words: *focus your thoughts.* When we learn to focus our thoughts during exercise we revisit the role our body plays in our life and begin to recognize it as a sacred vessel. Focusing our thoughts also keeps us in the present moment and allows us to bring in the elements of gratitude and joy into our movement experience. No matter what exercise we are doing, our ability to focus will make the difference between a purely physical workout and one that renews and refreshes our spirit as well.

The three general components of any well-rounded fitness program include strength, flexibility and cardiovascular exercises and these are the major areas that we will look at in relationship to adding spirit to your workout. In this chapter strength and flexibility are covered in depth along with suggested programs for scheduling these exercises into your busy day. Concluding the chapter is a *Bonus Boosters section* which touches upon additional exercises that can boost your awareness of the connection between body and spirit. Breathing and balance exercises are just two of the areas covered in this section.

While cardiovascular exercise can cover a wide range of activities, walking is probably the most accessible as well as the most popular form of this type of exercise. For this reason a large portion of Chapter Seven is devoted to demonstrating the many ways spirit can enhance your aerobic workout through walking. You will find an abundance of suggestions interwoven in the chapter that you can apply to any form of heart-pumping exercise. The chapter ends with a section on learning the language of the body and discovering insights into deeper dimensions of our physical form.

You will find help in putting it all together in the last chapter with the Seven Strategies for Success. With these strategies you will be well-equipped to embark on a magnificent journey of self-renewal. Now let's begin.

Strength and Flexibility

Strength training can do so much more than tone muscles. It can also give us an inner strength that unleashes our spirit, opens our heart and allows our mind to embrace a state of pure bliss. It can lead us to realize once more that life is indeed a celebration and an adventure; that it is full of discovery and opportunity. And sometimes it enables us to tap into the field of pure potentiality that rests within us.

I remember unexpectedly tapping into this field one day while taking care of my dad shortly before his passing. While he was strong and healthy for most of his life, the last month found him dependent upon a wheelchair with little use of his legs. Maneuvering him from the wheelchair to the commode was a huge undertaking, and was one task that was always left to the males of the family. But I was alone with dad one day when it became quite evident that the trip to the bathroom needed to be taken. He was almost twice my weight, and being inexperienced in these matters I knew that on a purely physical level this task was impossible. Yet I had no other choice than to do it. So defying all logic, I wheeled my dad to the bathroom, matter-of-factly evoking the help of the angels along the way. The transition was effortless. My dad felt like a feather and for minutes afterward I sat in amazement at the miracle that had happened. It was not my physical strength, but the inner strength, the tapping into the unlimited potential of the universe that allowed the transition to be smooth and easy for both of us. Physical strength is good, but when you add the dimension of spirit the impossible becomes the possible. You acquire a supernatural strength that can only be described as miraculous.

This chapter is all about using exercise to develop our inner as well as our outer strength. We can add this inner dimension to our workout by incorporating our knowledge of the chakras with focused attention on our thoughts and feelings during our exercise experience. To assist you in this effort I've included a "Thoughts to Ponder" section for each area of the body. This is an important part of the exercise that will help you connect with both your body and your spirit and bring a greater awareness to your exercise session. Aligning the body, mind and spirit in this way will allow the exercise session to be a holistic experience and a beautiful expression of life.

A Short Strength Training Primer

While the benefits of doing any type of strength or resistance training are plentiful, this area has been traditionally shunned by many women—until recently. Today women are beginning to recognize its importance, although many continue to feel intimidated or indifferent about following any type of strength training program. Part of the reason is that some aspects of how to begin, maintain, or enjoy an effective resistance training program remain a mystery to them. Some might even argue that enjoying strength training is about as conceivable as enjoying a trip to the dentist. But it is possible. It's all about changing your viewpoint.

Strength training, as well as movement in general, can be a wonderful opportunity to connect to the beauty of our spirit and allow the spirit to fully express itself in all its radiance. When we approach strength training with the intention of liberating our spirit, the benefits we receive from our workout increase exponentially. The exercise now becomes an occasion to cultivate qualities such as beauty, wisdom, harmony, inner strength, courage and peace. By focusing your attention on the inner qualities you wish to develop, you raise the vibration of the exercise and make it an exhilarating experience.

Strength training helps us connect once again to our own intrinsic power that we may have buried deep inside ourselves many years ago. A story I once heard about the training of elephants explains how easily this can happen. As the story goes, young elephants are initially chained to a pole with an extremely strong chain. As much as the young elephants try, they cannot move the pole or break themselves free from the chain. They learn that they are powerless. Paradoxically, as the elephant grows and becomes physically stronger, its spirit gradually becomes weaker and so does the chain that binds it. By the time the elephant is fully grown its spirit is crushed to the point where it no longer attempts to break free from the pole. A trainer knows this and will actually replace the sturdy chain with a simple rope. The idea that they are powerless has been ingrained so heavily in their brain that the older elephant fails to make even the feeblest attempt to break free. Like the elephant, many of us have been conditioned to think of ourselves as powerless and we no longer attempt to break free from any binds that have been placed on us. Through strength training we can reconnect to the strength of our spirit, release the binds that limit us and move forward in life with confidence and a renewed sense of self.

Whether you are doing strength training exercises for physical or spiritual development, there are some key principles to keep in mind in order to make your exercise an enjoyable and safe experience. Following these principles will ensure that both your body and spirit grow through pleasure not pain.

Principle #1: *Always warm up.* Whether you are working on strength training, stretching or cardiovascular exercises, it's always safe to warm up first. This increases blood flow to the muscle and also increases the body temperature, both of which reduce the chance of injury. Walking for about 10 minutes is an excellent warm-up.

Principle #2: *Perform the exercises SLOWLY.* This applies to both stretching and strength training. For stretching, hold the full-stretch position for at least 20–30 seconds without bouncing. For strength training, perform each exercise to the count of four. In other words, if you are performing a bicep curl, slowly count to four as you raise the weight, and slowly count to four as you lower it. Performing the exercises slowly helps us to be fully present with the exercise and also maximizes the results, both externally and internally.

Principle #3: *Never perform strength training exercises on the same muscle group two days in a row.* Improvement takes place during the rest phase. If there isn't any rest phase, the muscle will be overworked, the chance of injury will increase and results will be minimal.

Principle #4: *Always work the entire limb.* This pertains to work done with the arms and the legs. For example, if stretching or strengthening the quadriceps (front upper thigh muscles), it's important to do the same with the hamstrings (back of thigh muscles).

Failure to do this will result in muscle imbalances and greatly increase the risk of injury. Always think balance.

Principle #5: *Always stretch after strength training.* Many people understand the importance of stretching before strength training, but they fail to see the benefit of doing it after the workout. In fact, it's probably more important to stretch at the end of the workout than in the beginning. This is because the muscles contract and tighten up during strength training, so post-workout stretching will help to relax them and discourage muscle soreness from developing. When you are performing strength exercises on all the major muscles of the body, stretches can be done after each individual muscle group or at the end of your entire routine.

Principle #6: *Be totally in the NOW.* Focus your full attention on the exercise you are performing and how the body is responding to the movement. This will help you develop the ability to listen to your body and pay attention to what it is telling you. Dr. Christine Page once said that if we took our body to counseling, it would divorce us. We seldom are aware of the messages that the body is giving us. Learn to listen to the wisdom of the body. It may take some practice, but it is certainly well worth the effort.

Principle #7: *Remember that you are unique.* This principle is closely related to the previous one. While we are all composed of bone and muscle and fat and fluids, there are wide variations in each of these components. Your muscles, for example, can be composed of either fast-twitch or slow-twitch muscle fibers, or a combination of the two. The muscle fiber type which predominates in your muscle plays a major role in the physical results you receive from your training. A person who has a majority of fast-twitch muscle fibers will generally be able to gain more muscle definition than someone who has a majority of slow-twitch muscle fibers. Also, some people inherently have the ability to stretch farther than others. So the bottom line is not to compare yourself to others. If you pay attention to your own body, you will experience maximum satisfaction and results.

Principle #8: *Challenge yourself, but don't overdo it.* In strength training, a set represents a specific number of repetitions. For example, doing two sets of 10 repetitions means performing an exercise ten times, resting for about 20 seconds and performing another 10 repetitions. The weight you choose should bring you to comfortable fatigue after the first set. If you cannot feel any strain at all on your muscles after the first 10 repetitions, the weight you are working with is too light. If you cannot complete the first 10 repetitions through the entire range of motion, the weight you are using is too heavy. Choose a weight that taxes the muscles enough to increase strength, but does not overtax them to the point of excessive fatigue.

The amount of weight you use also depends on your goals. Using a heavier weight and performing less repetitions (such as 8 reps instead of 12) works more on muscular strength. Using a lighter weight and performing more repetitions (12 or 15 instead of 8) works more on muscular endurance. The easiest way to explain the difference between muscular strength and muscular endurance is to look at an example. Let's say you are reconstructing a flower bed and need to transfer a huge load of soil from a truck to your garden. The greater muscular strength you have, the more soil you will be able to carry with each trip. The greater your muscular endurance, the more trips you can make before you become tired. By performing ten repetitions during your workout you can touch on both muscular strength and muscular endurance. This strategy is commonly used for those new to the experience of strength training.

Following are strength training exercises that work the major muscles of the body. These exercises are designed to be a starting point for developing strength, communicating with the body and experiencing a new dimension of living in physical form. Who knows? They just might be a springboard that will lead you to explore the gift of movement at a deeper level.

The Exercises

The Legs

Wall squat with exercise ball. Lean against a wall with your back, placing an exercise ball on your back, just above the waist, between your back and the wall. Your feet should be hip-width apart and legs extended, with feet on the floor about three feet in front of you. Lower your upper body until the thighs are parallel to the floor. Make sure that the knees never extend over the toes. If you find they do on performing the first rep, extend your feet farther from the wall. Hold this position for five to 10 seconds. Slowly return to starting position. Work up to 2 sets of 10 repetitions.

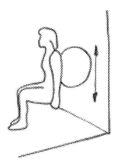

Stair climbing. This is a great exercise for both the legs and the cardiovascular system. To increase the strength benefits, do it *slowly* and *deliberately*. Instead of lifting your legs from one step to the next, push off with your foot. This engages many more muscles and increases the effectiveness of the exercise. For maximum results, go up two steps and down two steps for five minutes.

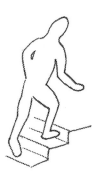

Seated isometric leg press. This is a great exercise for those who are not able to stand or have limited strength in their legs. While sitting in a firm chair, place both feet firmly on the ground. Align hips, shoulders, and head, keeping the spine erect. Press feet downward, as if digging your heels into the ground. Hold for five seconds, then release. Work up to 2 sets of 10 repetitions.

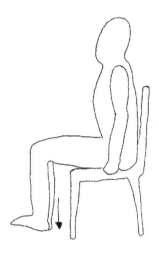

Alternate seated isometric leg press. This is another great exercise for those who are not able to stand. Maintain the same position as in the above exercise. This time, however, place both your hands on the right thigh. As you press down with your hands, lift the right thigh, against the resistance of your hands. Repeat with the left thigh. Work up to 2 sets of 10 repetitions.

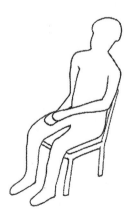

Thoughts to Ponder

As you strengthen your legs, tune in to your feelings. Do you feel secure and confident, comfortable in your body and connected to mother earth? Can you firmly step forward in life, with courage and self-assurance? Can you flow with the currents of life, easily and eagerly embracing change? Do you feel safe and supported by the universe? Can you confidently stand your ground? What does your body tell you?

Choose the feeling that you want to work on at this time, the feeling that draws your attention and pulls at your heart. It may be several. Then write your own affirmation that you can repeat as you exercise and feel the vibration of the affirmation awaken all the cells of your body. Sample affirmations follow.

I move forward with anticipation, excitement and expectancy.
I am free to move forward with joy and enthusiasm.
I step forward with courage and conviction.
I easily embrace change, moving into the future with grace and ease.
I eagerly look forward to all of life's adventures.
I move forward with confidence to do that which is mine to do.

Hamstring/calf stretch. Sit on a chair or bench with the left leg stretched out in front of you. Bend forward from the waist to a comfortable stretch, keeping the back straight and not rounding the shoulders. Breathe into the stretch. To involve the calf muscles, point the toes toward you. Hold the stretch for at least 20–30 seconds. Release, then repeat.

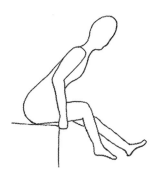

Quadriceps (upper thigh) stretch. Stand about one foot from a wall, with your right hand leaning against the wall for support. The right leg is straight, with knee slightly bent. Holding the left foot with your left hand, bend the left leg so that your left foot approaches your left buttocks. Hold the stretch for at least 20–30 seconds. Release, then repeat. Repeat with the other leg.

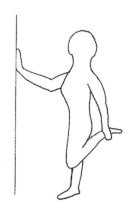

The Back

One-arm row. Start with the right leg kneeling on a bench and the upper body almost parallel to the bench, with shoulders slightly above the hips and the right hand supporting the upper body. The left leg is straight with a slight bend in the knee and the foot on the floor. Start with a dumbbell in the left hand, with the arm hanging straight down. Pull your left arm up from the elbow until the elbow is slightly above the core of the body. At the top of the motion, squeeze your back muscles. Slowly lower the dumbbell. Repeat with the other arm. Work up to 2 sets of 10 repetitions.

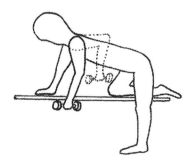

Lower back exercise. Kneel on the floor with upper body resting on an exercise ball, at about a 45 degree angle from the floor. Lift your shoulders back. You only need to move a few inches to feel the effect of this exercise. Note that the lower the ball is on your torso, the more challenging the exercise becomes. Work up to 2 sets of 10 repetitions.

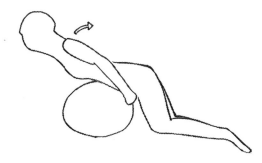

Thoughts to Ponder

As you work with the muscles in the back, focus on connecting with your emotions, honoring all your feelings. Only by owning our feelings and allowing them to fully express through us are we able to release those that do not serve us in our journey toward higher consciousness. Shapiro also reminds us that issues of survival, including the responsibility of earning a living, and carrying your own weight are connected to the back. Following are some suggested affirmations.

I am in the flow with all of life.
I am safe and feel supported by the universe.
I surrender to the flow of life, releasing all my fears.
As I let go of my fears, I know that all is in divine order.
I am free to live life with joy and enthusiasm and am supported by the universe.
I connect to the natural rhythm of life, embracing change with excitement and courage.

The Back Stretch. Sit on a chair with your feet flat on the floor about hip-width apart. Bend from the waist, slowly lowering your upper body as far as you can, until you are "hugging your knees" and hands are resting on the floor. Relax in this position, slightly arching your back, for at least 20–30 seconds. Slowly return to starting position beginning to lift your lower back first, then the middle and finally the upper back. Repeat as needed. This is a great exercise to do every hour when you find yourself sitting for an extended period of time.

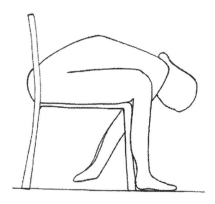

The Chest

The standard push-up. From starting position, place hands outside shoulder width with body straight. Lower body toward floor, inhaling as you lower. Exhale as you return to starting position. This exercise may also be done with the knees touching the floor. Work up to 2 sets of 10 repetitions.

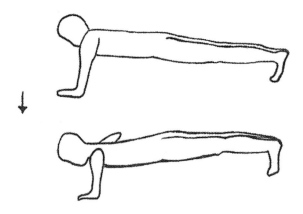

The bench press. Lie on a bench with knees bent, and a dumbbell in each hand, level with the chest. Exhale as you extend your hands straight above you, making sure you don't lock your elbows. Inhale as you bring the weights down to chest level. Work up to 2 sets of 10 repetitions.

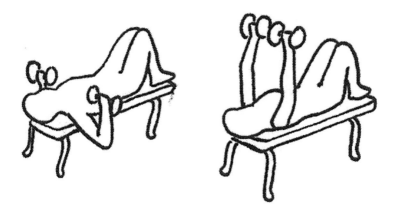

Thoughts to Ponder

While working on the chest area, focus on gratitude and appreciation for all the different parts of your body and begin to cultivate a deep feeling of love and acceptance toward it. This doesn't mean that you have no desire to improve your physical condition, but rather that you unconditionally accept your current state of health, knowing that care and attention will result in higher levels of wellness. Total acceptance allows you the freedom to move forward with anticipation and expectancy. Following are some sample affirmations.

I love and accept all parts of me.
I am grateful for the many ways my body serves me.
I move forward with anticipation and expectancy.
I enjoy who I am, and look forward to who I am becoming.
I am free to be me.

Pectoral stretch. Stand a few inches in front of an open door frame. Holding onto door frame with arms at shoulder level, lean forward until stretch is felt. Hold for 10 to 20 seconds, then return to starting position. Repeat.

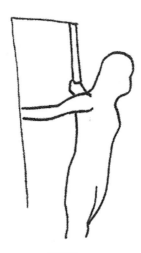

The Abdomen

The crunch. Lie on a carpeted or matted floor with knees bent and feet flat on the floor. Keeping head and neck in line with the spine, elevate shoulders and upper back toward the knees, keeping the low and middle back in touch with the floor. Exhale as you curl up, inhale as you return to the starting position. It is very important to make sure that all movements are smooth and you do not jerk. If this means that you only move a few inches, start at this point. With patience and proper form, you will be amazed at how quickly you will be able to advance.

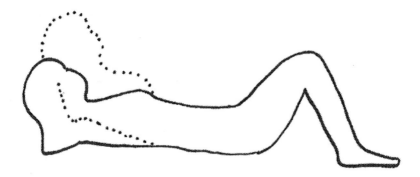

Seated reverse crunch. Some people find this exercise to be easier than the regular crunch. Begin by sitting on the floor with the spine erect, knees bent and feet flat on the floor. With arms stretched out in front of you, parallel to the floor, contract the abdominal muscles and slowly lean back toward the floor until the upper body is at a 45 degree angle to the ground. Hold for 5 seconds, then return to starting position. Exhale as you lean back, inhale as you return to the starting position. Begin with 10 repetitions and work up to 20.

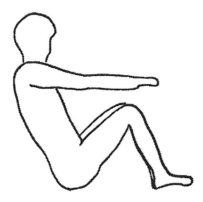

Seated twist. This area works the oblique muscles in the abdominal region. Begin with same position as the above exercise, then lean back a few inches. Fold arms in front of you so that the left hand is holding the right elbow and the right hand is holding the left elbow. Alternate rotating the upper body to the right, then to the left. Be sure to move only the torso. Perform 10 to 20 repetitions.

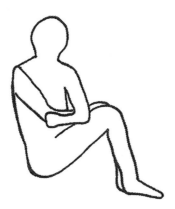

Thoughts to Ponder

While working on the abdominals, consider how you are nourished, both in terms of food and thought. Are you able to take in, assimilate and eliminate what is happening around you? Are you able to release what is no longer for your highest good? Do you follow your intuition or "gut feelings"? Below are some sample affirmations.

I release all that is not for my highest good.
I allow the perfection of life to flow through me.
I easily take in what nourishes my soul.
I follow my intuition with confidence.
I confidently accept all that greets me on my path, and trust the divine process.
I easily digest all that comes into my life.
I am safe in every situation and am supported by the universe.

Supine full-body stretch. Lie on your back on the floor with your legs straight and arms stretched out over your head. Make sure the small of the back is slightly arched. Stretch the entire body, holding the stretch for 10 to 20 seconds. Release and repeat.

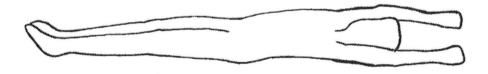

The Shoulders

Seated rear deltoid raise. Sit at the end of a chair or bench, "hugging" the knees with dumbbells in hands resting behind the ankles. Lift the dumbbells until arms are parallel to floor, keeping the arms slightly bent throughout the entire range of movement. Inhale as you lift, exhale as you lower the weight. Work up to 2 sets of 10 repetitions.

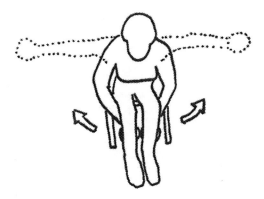

Seated lateral deltoid raise. Sit at the end of a chair or bench with the spine erect and arms resting at the sides. Lift the dumbbells, raising the arms at the sides until they reach shoulder height. Remember not to let the shoulders creep up, but only raise the arms. Inhale as you lift, exhale as you lower the weight. Work up to 2 sets of 10 repetitions.

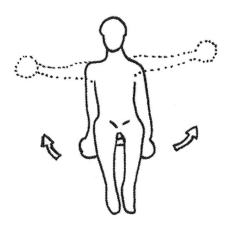

Alternating front deltoid raise. Stand with your spine erect, hands resting on the front thighs. Lift the right arm in front of body no higher than eye level. Make sure that the elbow joint is not locked. Slowly lower the arm to the starting position. Repeat with left arm. Work up to 2 sets of 10 repetitions.

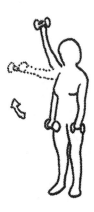

Thoughts to Ponder

While working on the shoulders, consider how you feel about your current level of responsibilities. Do you feel everything rests on your shoulders? Do you feel burdened with too many responsibilities? Are your responsibilities preventing you from doing what you really want? Some sample affirmations to turn around these feelings follow.

I easily release my burdens, knowing I have full support from the universe.
I handle my responsibilities with ease.
I easily connect with and express my feelings.
I embrace all my activities with love and laughter.
I enjoy what I do and I do it well.
My burdens are light and I handle them with ease.

Deltoid stretch. Stand with spine erect and feet shoulder-width apart and arms at your sides. Keeping arms straight, bring them behind you, interlacing fingers and pulling shoulder blades together. Hold for at least 10 seconds, then release and repeat.

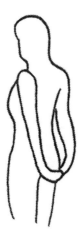

Posterior deltoid stretch. Sit with your spine erect and arms at your sides. Place right arm across the front of your body so that the right hand is resting on the left shoulder. With your left hand just above the right elbow, pull the right arm across the body until a stretch is felt. Turning your head to the right while stretching will enhance the stretch. Hold for 10 seconds, then release and repeat. Repeat with the opposite side of the body.

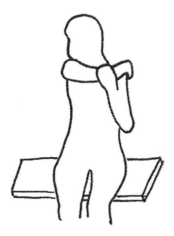

The Arms

Biceps curl. Stand erect with your feet shoulder-width apart, arms down at your sides, each holding a dumbbell. Slowly curl the right arm, bringing the dumbbell close to the right shoulder. Slowly lower the right arm. Repeat with the left arm. Caution: When performing this exercise, make sure that the only part of the body that is moving is the forearm. Do not "rock" the body. If this happens, it is an indication that the weight you are lifting is too heavy. Inhale as you curl the arm, exhale as you straighten it. Work up to 2 sets of 10 repetitions.

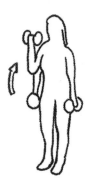

Standing one arm extension. Stand erect with feet shoulder-width apart, and arms at your sides. Begin with dumbbell in left hand, arm raised so that elbow is pointed toward ceiling and forearm is lowered behind back. Keeping upper arm stationary with right hand, slowly raise forearm to straight arm position. Return to starting position. Make sure that only your lower arm is moving, that your upper arm is remaining perfectly still. Repeat with the other arm. Work up to 2 sets of 10 repetitions.

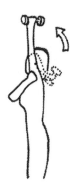

Thoughts to Ponder

While working on the arms, consider your deepest feelings. Can you take in and give out nourishment and love with grace and ease? Do you nurture yourself and others equally? Do you feel safe and secure in expressing all of your emotions? Can you embrace life with joy and enthusiasm? Shapiro shares with us that overdeveloped upper arm muscles may represent a desire to enter aggressively into activity while weak or thin upper arms can indicate a timid response to life and the inability to reach out and grasp hold of life. Following are some sample affirmations.

I eagerly embrace all that life has to offer.
I confidently respond to all situations in my life.
I easily give and receive love.
I openly share my deepest feelings.
I effortlessly express my innermost thoughts.

Biceps stretch. Stand erect with feet shoulder-width apart and arms at your sides. Keeping arms straight, bring them behind you, interlacing your fingers. Next, raise your hands toward the ceiling, holding the stretch for 10 to 20 seconds. Release and repeat.

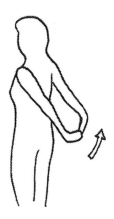

Triceps stretch. Stand erect with feet shoulder-width apart and arms at your sides. Keeping arms straight, bring them above the head, with fingertips pointing toward the ceiling. Bend left arm so that left hand is touching right shoulder. With right hand, pull left elbow behind the head until a stretch is felt. Hold for 10 to 20 seconds. Repeat on other side.

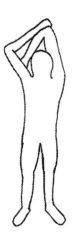

Scheduling for Strength

Implementing a strength training program is easy and effortless especially since there are so many ways you can schedule these exercises into your day. Three of these options are listed below. Choose the one that best fits into your lifestyle.

1. The Daily Approach. This plan involves a time commitment of 5 minutes, 5 days per week and focuses on one muscle or group of muscles per session.

DAY	MUSCLE AREA	EXERCISES
Monday	Legs	Wall squat with exercise ball Seated exercise leg press Hamstring/calf stretch Quadriceps stretch
Tuesday	Back/Chest	One-arm row Lower back exercise Standard push-up Bench press Pectoral stretch Back stretch
Wednesday	Shoulders	Seated rear deltoid raise Seated lateral deltoid raise Alternating front deltoid raise Deltoid stretch Posterior deltoid stretch
Thursday	Arms	Biceps curl Standing one-arm extension Biceps stretch Triceps stretch
Friday	Abdominals	Crunch Seated reverse crunch Seated twist Supine full body stretch

2. Split Body Approach. This plan involves a time commitment of 15 minutes, twice per week, and focuses on an entire section of the body per session.

DAY	MUSCLE AREA	EXERCISES
Tuesday	Legs, Abdominal, Back	Wall squat with exercise ball
		Stair climbing
		One-arm row
		Lower back exercise
		Crunch
		Seated reverse crunch
		Seated twist
		Hamstring/calf stretch
		Quadriceps stretch
		Back stretch
		Supine full body stretch
Thursday	Chest, Shoulders, Arms	Standard push-up
		Seated rear deltoid raise
		Seated lateral deltoid raise
		Alternating front deltoid raise
		Biceps curl
		One-arm extension
		Pectoral stretch
		Deltoid stretch
		Posterior deltoid stretch
		Biceps stretch
		Triceps stretch

3. Whole Body Approach. This plan involves a time commitment of 30–40 minutes, one day per week and includes all the major muscle groups of the body. Perform all the exercises listed in the split body approach. You may do all the strength exercises first and end with stretching.

Bonus Boosters

There are a few other exercises which are generally not included in any basic strength training program but which I believe are important in deepening the connection between the mind and the body. They help complete the total picture of what it means to be a spiritual being having a human experience. Working with these areas can boost your awareness about the amazing potential of the physical body.

The Neck

Neck exercises. Begin by sitting straight, spine erect and eyes looking straight ahead. Start by slowly lowering the head until the chin meets the chest. Next, slowly raise head until the chin is pointing to the ceiling. Return to starting position. Next, slowly turn head as far as you can to the left, keeping the shoulders square. Follow by slowly turning the head as far as you can to the right. Return to starting position. Next, slowly drop head to the left so that the left ear approaches the left shoulder. Make sure you do not lift the shoulder, but bring the ear down to meet it. Return to starting position. Next, slowly drop head to the right so that the right ear approaches the right shoulder. Return to starting position. Repeat five times. For variety, and more of a challenge, you can do all of the above exercises against resistance. While performing the exercises, resist with your hand either on the forehead or the side of the face. The key point to remember is to do all the exercises *slowly*. If any exercise brings you discomfort, stop immediately.

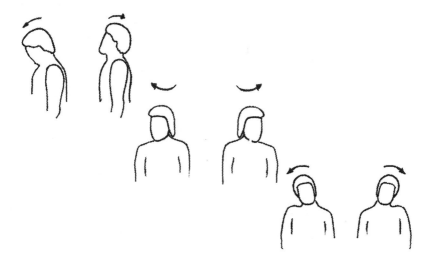

Thoughts to Ponder

When working with the neck area, place your attention on your ability to freely communicate your thoughts and emotions to others with truth and honesty. This is about speaking from the heart. This is about communicating with Source, asking through prayer, and listening through meditation. It's also about listening to others with full attention and an open mind. Some suggested affirmations are:

I easily speak my truth.
I clearly hear the voice of Spirit.
I am able to speak honestly and with love.
I am a good listener, open to the thoughts of others.
I open my heart and always speak with loving kindness.
I see all sides to the situations in my life.
I fully participate in life.

The Eyes

Figure Eight eye exercises. Sit in a chair with your spine erect and head straight. Imagine a figure eight, on its side, in front of your eyes. Moving only your eyeballs and keeping your head straight, trace the figure eight beginning at the center point and going up and to the right. This exercise will bring balance to the third eye and increase your ability to focus.

Alternative eye exercises. Sit in a chair with your spine erect, and head straight. Moving only your eyeballs and keeping your head still, slowly look upward then downward. Bring your focus back to center, looking straight ahead. Next, still keeping your head still, slowly look to the far right, then to the far left. Bring your focus back to center. Next, slowly look to the upper right, then to the lower left. Bring your focus back to center. Follow this by slowly looking to the upper left, then to the lower right. Bring your focus back to center. Finally, close your eyes and relax in the darkness.

Thoughts to Ponder

In working with the eyes, our thoughts center on releasing attachment to matter and desires of the ego. We see beyond the material world and begin to see Reality with a capital "R." From the "big picture" perspective, we clearly see and understand the law of cause and effect and the perfection of the universe. We also begin to recognize and rely on our own intuitive wisdom.

I see and think clearly.
I see the perfection in my life.
I see the perfection in the world around me.
I trust my intuition.
I rely on my own inner wisdom.
I eagerly move forward, illuminated by my higher vision.

Vocal exercises. These exercises actually have the capacity to stimulate the entire body, not only the throat area. This ability is based on the principle of vibration. Sound is vibration, and since every cell in our body responds to vibration, it responds to sound. Remember that the neck area is governed by the throat chakra and the sound for the throat chakra is "ee" like in seek. Slowly chanting this sound repeatedly for at least one minute, stimulates this chakra. It has also been said that chanting the vowels of the alphabet is a good exercise to stimulate the entire body. Try either one and notice how the body feels. Usually the body will feel very calm and relaxed.

Balance

Balance is an important part of living. Everyday our cells work to keep a balance within the body through homeostasis. Balancing work and family responsibilities with fun and pleasure is necessary to keep stress and illness at bay. If our muscles are not balanced, the risk of injury increases dramatically. One of the most popular and effective exercises for maintaining and improving balance is the practice of t'ai chi. By learning to balance the contraction and relaxation of our muscles we learn to move and shift our body weight in a graceful, flowing manner. In many ways, on many levels, life is truly a balancing act.

In addition to the above examples, there is another aspect of balance that is instrumental to our health and well-being. It concerns our ability to feel comfortable in our surroundings and to be able to connect to our environment with a natural grace and ease. This aspect of balance involves the vestibular system.

The vestibular system consists of a network of receptors and neural elements located in the inner ear. This system works mainly with balance: up and down, side to side, back and forth. It helps us handle a rough plane ride, the wave motion on a ship, and elevator or escalator rides. It also helps us with walking. When we walk or run, our head is usually pitched downward by approximately 30 degrees. This allows the line of sight to be directed a few meters in front of the feet. This position causes some of the components of the vestibular system to be parallel with the earth horizontally and perpendicular to gravity, and provides us with a comfortable orientation to our surroundings so that we can step forward with confidence, sure of the ground in front of us. A highly efficient vestibular system helps us feel at one with the earth and with creation. We feel comfortable and relaxed in our surroundings. We can easily adjust to environmental changes, and when the surface we are walking on changes, we alter our steps accordingly.

Sharon Heller explains in *too loud, too bright, too fast, too tight* that the vestibular nuclei start to develop nine weeks after conception and begin to function between the 10th or 11th week; by the fifth month in utero they are well developed. This makes sense when you think about the environment in which a fetus develops. Its host, the mother, may be standing, sitting, laying, twisting, bending, walking, and even jumping. Through all of this movement and change in orientation, the fetus needs to feel comfortable. And the vestibular system provides this comfort. In fact, it is the movement of the mother which actually stimulates the development of the vestibular system, allowing the fetus to relax whether it is upright, on its side, or even inverted. So movement is crucial for this system to develop properly. The fetus knows the importance of this movement, and that is why, when the mother rests, the fetus seems to move more. It appears to be trying to compensate for the inactivity of the mother.

But movement is not only important before birth. If we want to function comfortably in a changing world and maintain our balance as we age, our vestibular system needs to be stimulated. Any whole body action, such as walking, can stimulate the vestibular system, allow us to maintain a comfortable orientation with our surroundings and increase our body awareness. A balance ball, however, can exponentially boost these results. According to Heller, "Rolling back and forth on your belly on a large exercise ball for 15 minutes sets off a vestibular pow that has a long-lasting effect."

If you want to test your ability to stay in balance and get an idea of how well you orientate to your surroundings, there is a simple test that you can take. It's fun to do, and often very enlightening. Begin by standing with your body perpendicular to a wall. Make sure you have a clear path to walk along the wall for several yards. Standing erect, walk forward, placing the left foot in front of the right, with the left heel touching the right toes. Walk toe-to-heel for the length of the wall, always keeping your eyes looking forward. Only touch the wall for support if you become unbalanced. When you get to the end of the wall, turn around and walk back to your starting position.

For most people this first part of the exercise is easy and effortless. However, the next part leave many of them surprised. Do the exercise again, but this time close your eyes. Can you still walk smoothly, toe to heel, for a few yards without getting unbalanced or touching the wall? If not, roll on a balance ball for a few minutes and test yourself again. The results are sure to be very revealing.

The importance of feeling balanced within your body has not escaped the awareness of the medical profession. Chiropractors, occupational and physical therapy specialists, pain specialists, holistic health educators and energy medicine practitioners have used specialized machines called sensory integrative machines to develop and refine this skill in their patients. One of the pioneers in the field of sensory integration is Dr. Larry Shultz. According to Shultz, as the fetus grows it develops specific receptors that are designed to sense changes in motion so that it feels comfortable in its fluid environment. These receptors are located throughout the body and are in constant communication with the brain, both sending and receiving signals. Sensory integration machines provide wave-like motion therapy that stimulates these receptors and results in a heightened sense of balance for the participant.

My experience with this machine was an incredible revelation. It allowed me to fine tune the interaction between the nervous system and muscular contraction and relaxation on a very discrete and precise level so that I became intimately aware of the smallest change in the position of my body. Every move you make is reflected and magnified by the movement of the machine, so in some ways it acts like a huge biofeedback instrument. When you learn through this machine to move the muscles in a fluid manner, you achieve a superior level of balance that allows you to glide from one movement to the next with a smoothness that makes the experience feel like a dance with the divine. It teaches you to not only feel balanced within yourself, but also to feel at one with the flowing energy of the universe. It is a wonderful, euphoric experience. Whether you have an opportunity to experience a session on a sophisticated machine, or simply use a balance ball, performing exercises that stimulate your vestibular system and work on balance will help bring a new level of symmetry to your muscles and your life.

Balance ball exercise: Position yourself on your stomach on a balance ball with legs extended and toes touching the floor. Arms are bent so that the palms of your hands are touching the floor. With your arms roll yourself forward so that the ball is now between your hips and knees. Roll back to starting position. Repeat for 10 minutes.

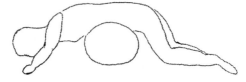

The Breath

Our breath is what gives us life. We can live days without food or water, but only minutes without breathing. Though it is so vital to our existence, it is often taken for granted. Gay Hendricks tells us in *Conscious Breathing* that each day we inhale and exhale approximately twenty thousand times. In our lifetime we will breathe in and out approximately a hundred million times. Yet, for the most part, this is all done without a single conscious thought.

Changing the way we breathe can lead to dramatic changes in our health. Jillian Hessel explains in *Pilates Basics* that "Shallow breathing can be the beginning of a downward spiral of health problems. It impairs mental acuity, causes headaches, increases anxiety, hampers the immune system, slows circulation, and decreases muscle and organ function." Compare this to the benefits of powerful breathing which include increasing the efficiency of the internal organs, stimulating circulation, improving digestion, reducing stress, enhancing relaxation and strengthening the abdominal muscles.

The lungs are a fascinating organ. If you spread out all four lobes of the lungs, they would easily cover the entire area of a basketball court. It is interesting to note that less than a tenth of a liter of blood flows through the top of the lungs every minute. Contrast this to two-thirds of a liter which passes through the middle part of the lungs, and over a full liter which circulates through the bottom of the lungs. It is clear to see the benefits to taking full, deep breaths. One great exercise is to focus on the breath several times throughout the day, consciously making each breath deep and powerful. Following are a few more exercises.

Deep abdominal breathing. This is something I tell my clients to do on a daily basis. Spending at least two minutes in the morning and two minutes in the evening focusing on slow, deep abdominal breathing energizes the body, calms the mind and soothes the spirit. "Breathing is how spirit moves through matter; it's our most down-home religious movement," shares Gabrielle Roth in *Sweat Your Prayers*. To enhance the spiritual benefits of breathing, imagine each breath laced with molecules of love and compassion. Follow the path of the breath, and feel that love and compassion sink into every cell of your body. Make sure that you breathe deep into the abdomen.

Alternate Nostril Breathing. Place the right thumb on the right nostril. Inhale slowly through the left nostril. Block the left nostril with your index finger; then lift the thumb and exhale slowly through the right nostril. Inhale through the right nostril. Then block the right nostril while lifting the index finger and exhale through the left nostril. Inhale through the left nostril then block the left nostril while lifting the thumb and exhale through the right. Repeat for two minutes. In *Conscious Breathing*, Hendricks tells us that alternate nostril breathing balances the brain. This is because the left nostril is connected to the right side of the brain and the right nostril is connected to the left side. He also shares that this exercise improves mood, refreshes the body and sharpens the mind.

The Mind and Meditation

You may think that meditation is a strange topic to include in a chapter on exercise, but looking at it from another perspective, it really makes a lot of sense. Meditation is actually a great exercise for the brain. It helps clear the brain of clutter, making communicating with the body much easier. Judith has another slant on the practice of meditation and its importance in clearing the mind. She shares: "We take it for granted that we need to take showers, clean our house and wash our clothes. Yet the mind and its thoughts need cleansing as much as our bodies. While few of us would consider eating dinner on yesterday's dirty dishes, we think nothing of tackling our problems with yesterday's cluttered mind."

A wonderful description of the benefits to be gained from meditation and decluttering the mind comes from Eckhart Tolle. In *The Power of Now*, Tolle states: "As you go more deeply into this realm of no-mind, as it is sometimes called in the East, you realize the state of pure consciousness. In that state, you feel your own presence with such intensity and such joy that all thinking, all emotions, your physical body, as well as the whole external world become relatively insignificant in comparison to it." To feel your own presence with such intensity and joy that all problems seem to drift away is certainly a great reason for calming the mind and clearing out the clutter.

The brain is governed by the crown chakra and represents our connection to spirit by whatever name we call it: higher power, God, Universal Source, Divine Source. It reflects our capacity to allow our spirituality to become an integral part of our physical life. It represents awakening, union with the higher self, and the fulfillment of our true destiny.

The purpose of meditation is to quiet the mind, release attachment to the physical and connect to your inner spirit. It's about listening to that spirit. There are about as many different ways to meditate as they are people who meditate. You might want to experiment and see what method works for you.

Breath meditation. One way for beginners to learn to meditate is to focus on the breath. Make sure that you are in a quiet room where you will not be disturbed. You may want to play a meditation CD or tape that includes music only. Close your eyes and focus on the breath. Whenever your thoughts wander, simply acknowledge them and return to the breath. You may also want to imagine breathing in love and exhaling all cares and concerns. The more you practice, the easier it will become to focus on the breath and release other thoughts. Begin with five minutes and work your way up to 20 minutes or longer.

Mantra meditation. Begin by sitting in a quiet room where you will not be disturbed. You may want to play a meditation CD or tape that includes music only. Repeat, in your mind, any word or phrase that helps you relax. An example would be thinking "peace" as you inhale and "love" as you exhale. You can also think "I am" on the inhalation, and "love" or "peace" on the exhalation. It doesn't matter what word or phrase you repeat in your mind. What matters is that it is simple and soothing.

Walking meditation. The purpose of walking meditation is to feel a connection to everything around you; to feel a oneness with all of existence and to open up to, and be aware of, your expanded self. Walk at a comfortable pace, being conscious of every step you take. Be aware of what your feet feel like when they touch the ground, how your breathing feels as it takes in fresh oxygen and releases carbon dioxide, how your back and shoulders feel, and how your legs feel as they carry you forward. Notice everything around you. Just observe, making no judgments. You will be amazed at how relaxing a walking meditation can be.

Thoughts to Ponder

In working in this area, we focus on freeing ourselves of the distractions of living in the material and connecting, instead, to our own limitless nature. It is here that we seek to understand our true essence, our oneness with All That Is. This is an area of expansion, where there is full awareness that all is one, and there is no separation or duality. And since we are one with all, it is here that we realize that what we do and what we think affects the world around us. Suggested affirmations for this area are:

I am at peace.
I am.
I am divine consciousness.
I am connected to All That Is.

The options for adding these exercises into your workout routine are virtually limitless and can depend upon your need as well as your desire. If you find yourself regularly in a frantic and stressful environment, meditation exercises may be a top priority. If you do a lot of desk work or driving, practicing the neck exercises on a regular basis would probably be beneficial. If you have a challenge with speaking your truth, and find that you say *yes* too often when you really wanted to say *no,* the vocal exercises may give you the strength to speak what is in your heart. Working with the eyes helps us to see better on many levels. And for many of us, improving our balance and breathing keeps us centered both physically and emotionally.

Determine what areas, if any, are important to you now and schedule five minutes, a few times per week, to practice the exercise that stimulates that area.

Be consistent and within a month or two, sometimes even a week or two, you will begin to observe a change in your body as well as your life. The change may be small at first but it will be a solid beginning to experiencing the lasting benefits of taking a proactive step to better health and well-being.

Doing your best

Exercise does so much more than strengthen your body. It gives you the inner strength to fully express who you are and to embrace all that life has to offer. It gives you the courage to move forward with confidence and a sense of adventure. It allows you to totally engage in life with excitement and expectancy. It sends the message to the universe that you intend to use every fiber of your being to wholly participate in life on this planet. Only by making these claims for yourself, will life reciprocate and provide you with experiences beyond your wildest dreams. Crystal Andrus emphasizes this point in *Simply Woman* when she says, "If you don't demand the most of yourself, you can never demand it out of life; and life only gives us what we demand of it."

This statement made by Andrus became clear to me when I finished a mini-triathlon a number of years ago. The event consisted of a one-half mile swim, a 20-mile bike ride, and a 3-mile jog. For my fitness ability at the time, this combination was short enough to be fun yet long enough to be challenging. And since I didn't learn to swim until age 30, it also represented a milestone for me. It would be another confirmation of my transition from an inactive to active life-style.

The weather was perfect and so was the water temperature. I felt nervous, confident and excited all at the same time. If I could make it through the swimming portion, I knew I could finish the race. I was right. I had successfully completed the swim, the bike ride and most of the run. The finish line was only about 50 yards away. I was comfortably jogging behind a woman with the pleasant thoughts of success filling my mind. When the woman decreased her speed, so did I. I had plenty of energy and could have easily passed her, but instead I slowed down and literally coasted across the finish line. My goal was to finish the race and I achieved my goal. I was a finisher.

It wasn't until later that I found out the woman I had followed through the finish line was in my age group. She placed third in the age group and received a medal for her efforts. If I would have done my best, I would have received that medal. But I slacked off, I coasted, and in the process missed out on one of life's sweet rewards. I found out that day that coasting may seem like a good idea at the time, but in the long run it prevents you from experiencing all that life has to offer. Not receiving the medal was not as important as the message behind it. To me it seemed to say that you never know what gifts life has waiting for you unless you participate fully in every moment. Give life your best and the same will be returned to you.

"Come to the edge.
We might fall.
Come to the edge.
It's too high!
Come to the edge.
And they came.
And he pushed.
And they flew."
—Christopher Logue

CHAPTER 7

▼

THE WISDOM OF
WALKING

"Imagine if, just for one day, everyone in the world tried to be the best person they could be."

—Crystal Andrus

Some of the great minds of all time engaged in walking on a regular basis. Einstein walked, and so did Socrates. Perhaps this is because walking not only promotes a healthy body, it also encourages clear thinking as well. And it is the perfect exercise to connect to the world around you—if you do it mindfully. Danny Dreyer, ultra marathoner and author of *Chi Walking—Mindful Walking* states that "By approaching a walk in a mindful way, every session brings new insights and challenges." Walking mindfully elevates the activity from a mere physical exercise to soulful experience. This has been my experience on many occasions.

I remember recently walking early one morning at a small park near my home. It was a beautiful, sunny morning with the newness of the day still unfolding. I was training for a race and my walk that morning was brisk when I noticed an elderly man some distance ahead of me step off the path. As I approached him, it became clear that he had interrupted his walk to pick some wild berries that grew a few yards away from the path. I couldn't help but think about that message. In the journey of life, don't forget to stop and take in all the sweetness life has to offer. The point, after all, is not to get to the end of it as fast as you can, but to enjoy every minute of the ride. I made a point that day to take in all the sweetness I could.

Another insight came while I was walking at a similar park a few miles away. While nestled in the middle of a city, the park held the ambience of the country. Much of the park consisted of woods with a river running through it. It was the home of deer, fox, huge turtles, and tons of birds and squirrels. As I was walking, I felt the beauty and serenity of nature fill my soul, with each step anchoring a comforting peace into the cells of my body. It was a perfect morning. Then it occurred to me. Some of the trees were old, some had bare branches, and some had limbs that were cracked. Some trees were growing straight and some had bends and curves in their trunks. And it all looked beautiful. There was perfection in the imperfection.

There are many reasons why walking in nature is so relaxing, the least of which is the opportunity it affords us to connect with the natural rhythm of life. This is a gentle, flowing rhythm that speaks to the soul and permits the illusions of the world to drift away. There are no demands, deadlines, expectations or judgments in nature. There is only life fully expressing itself in all its grandeur. The beauty of the wildflowers, the grace of the birds and butterflies flying around us and the playfulness of the squirrels all touch our heart. Nature is existence in its purest form. And when we are in nature we seem to, for that period of time, take on its qualities. We become calm and carefree. We sense a richness and expansiveness in nature that opens our heart, expands our mind, and lifts our spirit. We recognize that we do live in a loving, exquisite universe. Whether it's a stroll by the ocean, a jog in the park or a walk around the block, walking outdoors is a wonderful gift that delights all of our senses and recharges our entire being. It revitalizes us like nothing else can.

Nature has its own vibration, and it is this vibration that speaks to our own natural rhythm enticing us to fall in step with the pulse of life. Technology often tempts us to swim against the current of nature. We push ourselves to do more and to do it faster even though our body, mind and spirit may cry for relief from a self-imposed hectic pace. Walking in nature allows us to synchronize our vibration with the vibration of the earth around us. We release the need to make things happen on our time schedule and learn to connect with the timing of nature. It is in this connection that we find peace.

Walking in nature also allows us to see the bigger picture. Somehow connecting with the trees, plants, rocks and chipmunks also permits us to connect to the larger circle of life. Any problem we may be struggling with shrinks under the open skies, and we return home refreshed and comforted. There is a plaque in my home that clearly expresses these sentiments with the following words: "When it was time, the tree came to rest on the forest floor and slowly gave itself back to the earth from which young saplings sprang anew." Nature seems to remind us that we are all part of a miraculous and sacred circle of life.

When we walk among the trees, under the stars or surrounded by the birds and butterflies, we find it much easier to release the stresses of the day and turn our thoughts inward. These thoughts can be both personal and profound and often leave us with a new and enlightened perspective. Thomas Armstrong, author of *The Human Odyssey,* shares that whenever "we choose to gaze inwardly, we can be sure that our contemplations will enrich us by bringing insight, tranquility, or even a new sense of identity into our lives." Nature gives us the opportunity to grow in so many ways through our inward reflections. It's almost as if we are recreating ourselves with every step we take.

With nature surrounding us as we walk it becomes so easy to recognize the miracle of our existence. We can see life unfold as we carefully and consciously step forward into a new way of being. I'm always amazed to see flowers and new growth spring up between cracks in cement on sidewalks and even expressways. It certainly speaks volumes about the resilience of life and demonstrates to us that growth is possible even in the most adverse conditions.

Walking is a universal form of movement that gives us the perfect opportunity to explore how we walk through life in general. Jamie Sams and David Carson pose the following questions in *Medicine Cards:* "What words would describe the way you move through both the material and spiritual worlds? In the final analysis, is your movement compatible with your greatest desires and goals?" Thinking about the answers to these questions has helped me on many days adjust my attitude and manner of being. For me the questions are a constant reminder to be conscious of the way I move through all areas of my life.

When the external surroundings don't seem to hold your interest, looking internally can be very rewarding. Many years ago Wayne Dyer spoke about his habit of thanking different parts of his body on a regular basis. It was the first time I ever heard this mentioned and the idea did seem a bit unusual. But since I have been known to do a number of unusual things in my lifetime, I decided to give it a try during my walks. I began to thank my legs, and my heart; my lungs and my kidneys; my eyes and my ears. Sometimes I would simply scan my entire body to really get in touch with how each part felt at the moment, and would always uncover tension or tightness that previously went unrecognized. There is deep wisdom in the body; some even say the wisdom of the universe is stored within our cells. In a movement such as walking we can begin to unlock the keys to this wisdom and discover what is hidden within.

You can also use walking as a time to express gratitude. And the list of what to be grateful for is endless—just think about it! Most likely you took a shower this morning and used soap, dried yourself off with a towel and brushed your teeth with the aid of a toothbrush and toothpaste. Think about all the people it took to bring those products to you. You could probably spend hours thinking about all the people that are involved in providing you with the comforts you enjoy. It could easily fill up your walking time—even if you were walking a marathon!

Sending thanks and gratitude out to others in this way is also a great game to play with kids. Ask them to think about all the people it took to provide them with their favorite toy or game. This not only teaches them about giving thanks, it also shows them how interdependent we are upon each other.

Along the same lines, I sometimes think about all the things that are going right for me—and there are many things here as well. Today, electricity was available whenever I needed it. The stove worked perfectly when I cooked my breakfast. I was able to drive to one of my favorite parks in a car that afforded me a smooth and comfortable ride. My computer allowed me to easily connect to friends across the nation. The telephone was functioning without any problems. Life was definitely working in my favor.

One person who definitely embraces a positive attitude toward life is Rob Brezsny, author of *Pronoia Is the Antidote for Paranoia.* Brezsny explains that pronoia was first coined by Grateful Dead lyricist John Perry Barlow and is defined as being "the opposite of paranoia." A pronoiac, therefore, is "someone who believes that the world is conspiring to shower him or her with blessings." What a great perspective!

In his book, Brezsny states that even though 99% of our day may have gone right, many of us have a tendency to focus on that 1% that didn't. To begin with, we wake up in the morning feeling refreshed and coherent even though we literally have been unconscious for about six to eight hours. We may have hot running water for a shower, comfortable clothes to put on and food to eat. Yet if we discover that our car has a flat tire, we immediately complain about the difficulties of life. The tragedy is that we often allow a tiny mishap to set the stage for our entire day. The truth is we can permit a challenge to disrupt our peace and pleasure or we can decide that our day will be a glorious and wonderful experience. Remember, as you declare it, so shall it be.

Your walking experience can be whatever you want it to be. The possibilities are endless. Thanks to portable electronics, you can walk while you listen to a comforting CD, a mystery novel, a foreign language lesson, or the favorite hits of the 60's. While we talk a lot about connecting to your body, sometimes you just need to escape for a few minutes and focus on something different. Honor your feelings. If you need to blow off steam, a comforting CD might not be the right choice. You want something with a strong beat that will allow you to forcefully walk forward releasing any anger or resentment with each step. If you're feeling a bit down, you may want to listen to something inspiring. Follow your gut and make your walk whatever you need at the moment.

Sometimes your walk or jog is filled with an unexpected treasure. I remember a marathon that I race-walked in Alaska to raise funds for the Leukemia Association. This was the first marathon that I had prepared for in five years and, because of complications, I hadn't been able to adhere to my training schedule. So I asked my friends in a prayer circle to see me completing the race "with a spring in my step, a smile on my face, and joy in my heart." At around mile 15 of the race, the course took us over a wooden "swing" bridge that traversed a little stream. As I crossed the bridge, a runner from behind commented to me: "Doesn't that put a spring in your step!" Remembering my earlier prayer request to my friends, the comment warmed my heart. Around mile 18 the course curved around a breath-taking scene of a valley and mountains. Another runner shared with me as he passed: "Doesn't that put a smile on your face!" This sent a tingling sensation through my entire body. Both runners had used the exact words I used in my earlier request. I knew then that I had the support of the universe with me. I was in such a euphoric state that I don't remember if another runner said anything about joy in the heart, but I know that's exactly what I felt when I crossed the finish line.

One of the most delightful benefits about walking is the opportunity to participate in fun runs. For those like me who have never participated in group or team sports, fun runs are an uplifting experience. These races can range from distances of 3 miles to 10 miles and are a great way to spice up your exercise program. Just imagine it. Police stop traffic just for you. Dozens of volunteers get up early in the morning and set up tables covered with cups of water just so they can hand one to you as you walk by. Hundreds of spectators come to cheer you on. And as you cross the finish line, a selection of food is available for you to enjoy. Many times there is an after-race party with music, raffles, and a variety of activities. All of this is organized to recognize you for the effort you put into your training and to celebrate and honor you for walking the distance. What a life-affirming experience!

Occasionally, participating in such an event can lead to additional rewards. One year my husband was competing in a triathlon and I went along for emotional support. I was heavy into jogging at the time and planned only on being a spectator. When we arrived at the event, I noticed that an 8-mile race was scheduled simultaneously and decided on-the-spot to participate in it. I knew I would finish in plenty of time to greet my husband as he completed his race.

The course circled around a charming little lake with giant trees providing shade along the path. During the race I began talking with one woman who ran about the same pace as I did. We kept each other company for about five miles when I suddenly realized that I was running slower than usual. My previous experience about not doing my best flashed in my mind and I was determined not to let that happen again. With a few parting remarks to my running partner, I picked up my speed and ran my own race. About two miles later as I rounded a bend in the road, I heard a race official speak into his phone that the first female had just come into view. He was talking about me! His words spurred me on to keep my lead and accomplish something I never would have imagined in my wildest dream. I became the first female to cross the finish line, and received a trophy for my efforts. I still smile when I think about the event because I also finished second to the last in the female category. You figure it out.

Signing up to participate in a fun run is also a great way to ensure consistency in your walking program, especially if you are doing the run for charity or a special cause. Telling others you are walking for a larger purpose often keeps obligations from encroaching on your training walks. The family suddenly agrees to fend for themselves at dinner and someone volunteers to take the kids to their team practice so that you can train. After all, you are doing it for a bigger cause. When you really don't feel like walking, thinking about the charity can inspire you to overcome your apathy and put on your walking shoes. Sometimes all you need is a short-term goal, like participating in a fun run, to get you started on a new path to making a major lifestyle change. A sample walking program that will prepare you to complete a 3-mile fun run can be found in the appendix.

Chopra reminds us that "Reading has an effect at the level of thinking; feeling and doing have to be touched if any change is to take place." Walking is a great way to begin to do something to form a new relationship with your body and with the world. Every step you take brings you closer to experiencing more joy and peace and love on this journey called life. Embrace the journey.

Learning the Language of the Body

Walking is also the perfect time to deepen your connection to your body by talk-ing—and listening—to it. While the following exercise was developed to be implemented in a sitting or lying position, it can easily be adapted to perform during a walk. Just make sure that you don't close your eyes!

Talking to the body exercise. Begin by sitting or lying in a comfortable posi-tion, in a place where you can be alone. Close your eyes and take three deep breaths. If soothing music helps you to relax, put on your favorite CD. Slowly scan your entire body, from the tips of the toes to the top of your head. It doesn't matter if you begin with the head or the feet; what matters is that you do this exercise slowly and consciously. Focus on how each area of the body feels. Are your muscles tight? Is your breathing relaxed? Does your back feel comfortable? Any discomfort that you feel is a message from the body. The message may be to move to a more comfortable position or to look into the pain that radiates from a particular spot. Discomfort is one way the body talks to you. It is telling you that changes are necessary if you want to feel better.

Notice that talking to the body begins with listening. After you have scanned the entire body and noted areas of concern, give thanks to the different parts of your body. Thank your lungs for taking in life-giving oxygen and releasing carbon dioxide. Thank the legs for taking you to so many wonderful places. Thank the immune system for handling all the "invaders" that daily enter your system. Slowly go through the entire body, thanking each system, each organ for the ser-vice they provide. Then take a few deep, cleansing breaths and see if you notice any difference in how you feel. Chances are that you will feel a new sense of vital-ity in every cell of your body.

Talking to the body is one of the most valuable exercises in this book. If it sounds a bit strange to you, begin by pretending. What do you think your stom-ach would say to you about all that it has to digest, both food and emotions? Does your back feel like it's supported? What would it take to make your shoul-ders and legs feel good? What does your body say about the amount of sleep it gets? Does it want to slow down? The questions are endless and the opportunity for learning something valuable is unlimited.

The biggest lesson I received from my body occurred when I first encountered my breathing challenges at the beginning of my fitness career. Plagued with constant congestion in my lungs and a cough that produced blood, I was desperate for relief. After consulting with a physician who specialized in respiratory illnesses and undergoing a series of tests, I found myself taking four prescription drugs four times a day. When following this routine for a month brought little change, the physician responded by prescribing more drugs. I responded by getting a second opinion from another professional—a spiritual nutritionist.

The interview with the nutritionist was an interesting and informative experience. Her examination included iridology (looking at the eyes) and an analysis of the soles of my feet. She shared that both of these areas on my body clearly suggested that my diet was responsible for much of my breathing problems. My body was sending me a message that the food I was eating needed to drastically change. The recommendation from the nutritionist was to eliminate all wheat and dairy and adopt a macrobiotic diet for six months. After following these recommendations for two weeks, 95% of my breathing problems disappeared. I was able to stop all medications except for the occasional use of an inhaler when exercising. I was overjoyed and overwhelmingly grateful to the nutritionist. In my haste to squelch through medications the uncomfortable symptoms emanating from my body, I almost missed an opportunity to understand the message that the symptoms were carrying. It was this understanding that empowered me to take control of my health and to begin to form a new relationship with my body.

One of the most insightful books on communicating with the body is *Your Body Speaks Your Mind* by Deb Shapiro. In this book, Shapiro presents detailed instructions on how to develop a dialogue with the body along with excellent exercises designed to initiate the process. Shapiro cautions that "Listening to your intuition, your feelings and your body is a gentle process of opening into awareness ... you have to first become internalized, with your attention facing inward rather than outward ... Patience is also needed here. You need patience to let your body speak to you ... You need patience with yourself in understanding your body's language." Indeed, communicating with the body is like learning a new language, and Shapiro's book is an excellent resource to guide you through the process.

The concept of talking to the body is also supported by Dr. John Upledger who founded the Upledger Institute in 1986, and is internationally known for his work in CranioSacral Therapy. Upledger explains in *Cell Talk* that the cells have consciousness and intelligence. Since tissues are made up of cells and organs are made up of tissues, and all the physiological systems of the body have cells as their root, the body is also conscious and intelligent. Upledger, therefore, theorized that we should be able to talk to it. Acting from this theory, he has talked to cells and parts of the body for years and shares some of his findings in *Cell Talk*. His dialoguing with cells has supplied us with a wealth of knowledge about the functioning and feelings of the human organism. Upledger shares that "Inside each of us is a wealth of genius that can be respectfully solicited to help us know ourselves." The key to obtaining this information is patience along with an open heart and mind.

In truth, talking to the body and getting in touch with the feelings that are stored in it may be a lot easier for some people than for others. This fact was confirmed to me when I took a required college class many years ago. One of the assignments for the class involved "dancing" the scene on a postcard that the teacher handed out to each student. I was completely mystified by the assignment and had positively no idea how to accomplish it. For two weeks I stared at the postcard and saw only buildings, a few trees and a little pond. No inspiration surfaced, not even a single step. In desperation I asked another student for help. After handing her the postcard, she gazed at it for a few seconds and immediately began to perform a beautiful, exquisite dance. Her movements were flowing, expressive and done with a deep passion as she moved gracefully across the floor. I was in awe of her artistic ability. Later she shared her secret. When I looked at the postcard I saw the physical structures. When she looked at it she saw the emotion and symbolism behind the structures. For her the trees and the buildings represented technology and nature in a type of ying/yang relationship, and the pond reflected the presence of a quiet peace among the other elements. I was definitely coming from my head and she was clearly coming from her heart.

Talking to the body is a heart experience. It is a feeling experience. For those like me who have a history of coming from the left brain and looking at things from an analytical viewpoint, learning to see through the feelings of the heart is a new experience. But this is exactly what is required in order to develop a deeper relationship with our body. If we continue to look at the human body as only a physical structure, then this is all we will see and experience. If we stretch our minds and recognize that the body represents so much more, that it is also a storehouse of every thought and emotion we've ever had, that it is the pathway to freeing our soul, that it is the source of much wisdom, then we unlock the door to another dimension of living. The information stored in our body has been accumulating since birth and is waiting for us to tap into it. By learning to listen with our heart, we can access this information and discover the intricate role our body plays in our health and happiness on this earthplane.

"Our deepest fear is not that we are inadequate. Our deepest fear is that we are powerful beyond measure. It is our light, not our darkness, that most frightens us. We ask ourselves, who am I to be brilliant, gorgeous, talented and fabulous? Actually, who are you <u>not </u>to be? You are a child of God. Your playing small doesn't serve the world."
—Nelson Mandela

CHAPTER 8

▼

MAKING IT HAPPEN

"Whatever the mind of man can conceive and believe, it can achieve."

—Napoleon Hill

Starting something new is always exciting. Enthusiasm is strong, expectations are high, and anticipation of positive results rules the mind. Continuing to be as excited on day 30 of a new program as on day one is another story. Oftentimes, boredom, discouragement and lack of interest seem to creep in and smother out those initial feelings of hope and expectation. Lifestyle changes do not happen automatically. It takes careful planning, and constantly adjusting the plan, to make a new habit permanent. Presented in this chapter are seven strategies that I have found to be pivotal for myself and others who I have worked with in making a proactive lifestyle a reality. Use these strategies as a guidepost to help you move forward with courage and conviction to a more self-empowering life filled with an abundance of health and overflowing with joy.

1. Know Your Starting Position

Imagine living in Michigan and logging onto the computer with the intention of getting directions to a friend's house in Wichita, Kansas. The computer asks you for your present location but you hesitate to put in your address. You feel that sharing any personal information on the internet is unsafe, so you put in the address of a friend in Panama City Beach, Florida. What then comes out of the computer are very specific directions for traveling from Panama City Beach to Wichita, and most likely would not be very helpful to you in Michigan.

Just as you need to convey your current physical location when seeking directions for traveling to another destination, you also need to know your current physical and emotional health in order to successfully move forward to a more vibrant, energetic life. Being aware of our current condition allows us to design a program that accommodates our tastes, builds on our strengths and minimizes our weaknesses.

While this sounds like common sense, many people prefer to skip this strategy. Why focus on an overweight body, sore joints, weak muscles or a tired spirit? The answer is not to focus, or criticize, or judge, but only to observe. Observation leads to knowledge and knowledge is power. Knowing our starting condition gives us the power to embrace our present state of health while focusing on a more active and vibrant future. When I attempted to train for a marathon after going many years without intense training, I was not aware of my starting condition. Examining my current physical state more closely enabled me to adjust my training and expectations and maximized my chance of success at my new goal.

Knowing your starting position can provide you with valuable information and can be done on many levels. You can do a deep analysis or a cursory examination. A good way to begin is to truthfully scan your entire body, noting what areas are calling for your attention. Be honest about your energy level, your weight (knowing the exact number of pounds is not necessary), your appetite or cravings, and any persistent pain or discomfort. You may also want to examine your emotional make-up. For example, if you are sensitive to the opinions of others, knowing this can be a clue for you to refrain from sharing your new commitment to a more proactive lifestyle with others who may be lacking the social skills of support and encouragement. Let your results speak for themselves. In addition to your body scan, you might find it helpful to undergo a complete physical by an allopathic physician or an alternative health care practitioner. Your options are many, so choose what feels right to you.

Sometimes observing our starting point helps us to appreciate our progress that might have otherwise gone undetected. Experiencing breathlessness after 30 minutes of walking when we have been following a walking program for four weeks may cause us to be discouraged. Yet, remembering that these same conditions occurred after only 10 minutes of activity a month ago when we started the program puts an entirely different perspective on the rate of progress. The more you are aware of your starting position, the more you will recognize the tremendous improvements that result from your commitment. And the more reasons you will have to celebrate!

2. Develop a Supportive Environment

Few people realize how significantly the environment influences them, or they don't believe that they can change it to any great degree. The truth is, your environment can be one of your greatest support systems to changing a lifestyle behavior, and sometimes some of the smallest changes can make a huge difference. The key is to be consciously aware of how your surroundings encourage or discourage any positive change. Once you fully understand the dynamics that are involved, change almost becomes automatic.

One of the most important places on the planet for each of us is our homes. Denise Linn reminds us in *Sacred Space* that our home is "not just a composite of materials thrown together for shelter and comfort. Every cubic centimeter, whether solid or seemingly empty space, is filed with infinite vibrating energy fields." These energy fields constantly interface with us and affect both our physical and emotional health. We all remember special places we have gone to where we have felt at peace and comforted and other places where we felt tension and stress. While we notice these differences in the places that we visit, many of us seldom think about how we feel about the energy of our homes. There are many things that we can do to increase the vibration of our homes and our environment in general. Following are some suggestions.

Things You Can Release

The very first step in raising the vibration of your home and making it more welcome is to declutter. There is no stepping around this first step. The more you clear out old things, the more you clear out old energy and allow a new, vibrant energy to come in its place. There are many ways you can do this. First, look to limit what you have. Do the things around you add to your life and make you feel good. If they don't make you feel good, then eliminate them. Newspapers and magazines are great examples. Sometimes just removing them from a room can free up the energy.

After reassessing the need for the newspapers and magazines, look at all the other objects in the room, those that are on the tables and shelves as well as those that are on the wall. How do you feel about each item that you see? Does it raise your energy or lower it? If you have no particular feeling at all, perhaps it needs to be removed. Do this exercise slowly and deliberately. What you will notice is that the items remaining take on a new energy that vibrates at a higher level. You will begin to feel lighter. Continue to weed out items, storing some and giving others away. If you find you really miss something that you have stored, you can always bring it back.

The next step is to have designated spots for items. This includes a box for toys, a rack for magazines, and a place for books or any craft you may be working on. Putting everything away, including clothes and shoes, also helps to free up energy. If you don't have enough drawers or closets to store everything, this may be a signal to do more recycling. Giving items to a local shelter does wonders for both lifting the spirits of you and your home.

Another energy booster is to limit the time the television is turned on, or if you are brave enough, eliminate it altogether. Barbara Marciniak tells us in *Earth* that television slows down our evolutionary process and limits us. She also suggests that it allows us to be passive rather than active, and suppresses our imagination. Marciniak challenges us to observe how we feel when we watch TV. This is good advice, and following it can be very enlightening. Is television an occasional form of entertainment for you or a regular means to escape reality? The next time you find yourself watching TV, check to see if you feel uplifted, energized, empowered or excited about the future? You may be surprised at what you discover.

If you do watch TV, watching with awareness may help nullify some of the potentially harmful effects of this mode of entertainment. At minimum, question what is presented before you and learn to discriminate fact from fiction. Whether it is a news program or commercials, be particularly aware of the underlying message that is offered, and consciously check to see if this message resonates with your belief system and is empowering. Any message that leaves you feeling depressed or discouraged about yourself or the future can undermine your desire to experience life to the fullest.

It is interesting to note that a large portion of television commercials are devoted to pills, medications, creams, or ointments designed to correct problems that occur when the body apparently malfunctions. These commercials may leave one with the belief that the body occasionally needs to be "fixed" and that the best way to fix it is to take the latest pharmaceutical. While a few of these commercials do mention the benefits of making healthy lifestyle choices, many simply suggest that relief can be easily and quickly obtained by taking the right drug.

Although this may be true, it misses a very important point. Health is a natural state of our body, and our body has the ability to always maintain optimal health in a supportive environment. A supportive environment is the key here. This means maintaining a balance between work and play, a healthy diet of whole foods, regular activity, and time to connect with nature. When pain or disease do manifest, it is not a malfunction but a signal from the body that our environment needs to be changed. Remember, our body is a messenger. It will always let us know when it can no longer handle the stresses we put upon it. When we silence the messenger by ingesting a drug without considering the message, we diminish the ability of the body to self-heal and our dependency on drugs increases. When we pay attention to what the body is telling us, and make the appropriate changes in our lifestyle, we empower ourselves and dramatically improve our health. While drugs are certainly lifesavers in many situations, an over-reliance may cause greater problems. It also diminishes the belief that we possess our own resources to manage our health. Our body has an amazing ability to correct any apparent malfunction. By being proactive and listening to the messages it sends us, we can experience incredible health throughout our entire life.

A final suggestion for elimination involves letting go of an excessive amount of responsibility. This includes responsibilities at work, home and the community. If you are sharing your living space with others, consider sharing the responsibility for keeping the place clean as well. What responsibilities can you delegate to others? What household tasks can be shared? Being solely responsible for a living space that involves others can feel like a huge burden on your shoulders. Finding ways to lighten that burden will result in a lighter and happier spirit.

Things You Can Add

One of the easiest ways to change the vibration of a room is through music. Sound is very powerful. Linn shares with us in *Sacred Space* that sound can "cleanse and clear the energies in your home … (and) speed up the vibratory rate in your home so that your home sings with light and life." Different types of music will produce different results. African drumming music can inspire creativity and strength while Bach music can soothe and relax. Experiment with the large variety of music that is available and see how each type affects your mood. Sometimes you may want the music to energize you and at others times you may want it to calm you. Whatever you desire, use music and enjoy the results.

Aromatherapy is another tool that can dramatically change the vibration of a room. Our sense of smell is the most powerful of our senses, and is linked closely to our emotions. How many times has a certain smell brought back memories of a previous time? It could be the smell of pipe tobacco or baked bread, a certain dish or even a distinctive leather smell. If it brings back a memory, it usually brings a strong emotion along with it.

Today we are fortunate enough to have a wide variety of scents available through essential oils. These oils can change the vibration of a room through the use of diffusers, sprays or candles. When working with scents, it is highly recommended to use natural essential oils rather than synthetic, commercially-made fragrances. In addition to the beautiful smell, essential oils carry with them the energy of the plant from which they were derived, bringing with them the energy of nature. This has the effect of bringing more life and vitality into a room. As with sound, different essential oils produce different effects on the environment. Lavender, for example, is very relaxing while lemon is uplifting and good for mental alertness. A list of some of the most common essential oils and their qualities can be found in the appendix.

Another way you can lift the vibration of a room is to add what I call "visual affirmations." This could be something as informal as a post-it note with the word *Believe* on it attached to your computer or as permanent as the word *Imagine* painted on a wall. As I look around my home office, I'm reminded about the importance affirmations have played in my personal and professional growth. When I first started college I had a poster clipped to my refrigerator of Snoopy running in one direction, Woodstock and his feathered friends running in the opposite direction, all above a caption that read, *I march to the beat of a different drummer.* This represented the beginning of my quest for self-discovery. As I worked to complete my second degree in exercise physiology and start my own wellness business with a partner, inspiration came from a poster that hung in my office. The poster displayed the silhouette of a woman running and the words, *I believe in me.* These words encouraged me to venture forward with courage and confidence. Many years later, an interest in energy medicine led to certification as a Healing Touch Practitioner and a healing practice. When this happened, the poster of the runner came down and a ceramic plaque with the words "*Follow Your Heart*" found a home on the credenza in my office. As my exploration of spirituality deepened, the phrase *Be the peace you want to see … Let joy and happiness prevail* was painted across the entire length of one of my office walls. And when I began to write about the connection between exercise and spirituality, the words *It's Time* were displayed inside a butterfly frame to remind me to continue to move forward. Affirmations have always been a source of encouragement for me and have made a huge difference in my ability to shift my perspective and my life. It's really impossible to underestimate their significance. Surround yourself with the affirmations that resonate with you and feel their message sink into every fiber of your being. They are guaranteed to change both you and your environment.

You may wonder why I've placed so much emphasis on the environment. The truth is, it makes a huge difference. In my experience delivering wellness programs to businesses, the corporate culture of the business was a significant factor in the program's success. If a company maintained a high stress level among its employees, lacked clear avenues of communication, or failed to respond to employee concerns, the effect of the wellness program was usually minimal. Employees found it very difficult to incorporate any positive lifestyle changes. Their working environment was anything but encouraging.

To the same degree, your home environment is instrumental to your success in adopting an active lifestyle. The time you spend assessing your living surroundings and making whatever changes you can, no matter how small, will maximize the success you will experience. Making these changes will, at best, be a strong support for you. At worst, making the changes will leave you with an environment that will be more relaxing, more peaceful, and more inviting to all who enter it.

3. Find the Intention that Inspires

After doing all that you can to make your environment supportive, the next step to embracing an active lifestyle is to focus on an intention that inspires you and transforms the flickering flame that lies within you into a blazing fire. Finding an intention that excites you and fills you with passion can change a mundane exercise session into an exciting adventure of discovery. It can make the difference between seeing exercise as a chore or experiencing it as a celebration. It is probably one of the most important keys to lifting exercise up from a purely physical workout to an opportunity for a spiritual awakening. What do you want to gain from spending more time exercising and connecting with your body? The more you can elucidate, and become excited about, exactly why you want to become more active, the greater your chances are of success. To make any change a reality, it's important to feel passionate about your purpose, to feel inspired to make it happen, and to emphatically believe that it is possible.

My journey into movement began with a voice deep inside telling me there was more to me than what I was experiencing. The voice was so strong, I couldn't ignore it. It was an unquenchable desire and in my heart I knew following it was the only choice I had. Listening to my inner voice and the message that I was so much more than I realized became my inspiration.

The power of inspiration is beautifully described by Patanjali, who wrote the following over 2,000 years ago: "When you are inspired by some great purpose, some extraordinary project, all your thoughts break their bonds, your mind transcends limitations, your consciousness expands in every direction, and you find yourself in a new, great, and wonderful world. Dormant forces, faculties, and talents become alive, and you discover yourself to be a greater person by far than you ever dreamed yourself to be."

From the above quote, it becomes clear that finding an intention that inspires can get us moving on early winter mornings when warm blankets are coaxing us to stay snuggled in bed. But how do we find that intention that inspires us about exercise if boredom and apathy have always been our experience in the past? The answer lies in looking at the intangible benefits of exercise and knowing the difference between extrinsic and intrinsic motivating factors.

Some of the traditional reasons given for becoming more active include losing weight, lowering blood pressure, decreasing cholesterol and increasing bone density. These are all examples of external or extrinsic motivating factors, and while they are certainly commendable objectives, external factors often lack the ability to sustain motivation in the long run. Let's look at weight loss as an example. A person sets up a goal to exercise in order to lose 20 pounds before a family wedding. Having a goal like this often keeps someone exercising regularly—at least for the time being. The challenge, though, is to continue exercising after the goal has been reached and the event has passed. Often, after the special event, the motivation is gone, and so is the exercise.

On the other hand, intrinsic motivating factors have the power to inspire and get you so excited about exercising that remaining sedentary is simply not an option. They are timeless, and often get stronger the longer you pursue them. Examples of intrinsic motivating factors include the desire to experience more joy in your life, the yearning to be surrounded with an abundance of beauty and harmony, or the longing to feel a deep sense of inner peace. Intrinsic desires are feelings that speak to your heart and soul. These feelings are the language of the spirit and propel you to embark on a pathway of unlimited possibilities. When your intention includes intrinsic desires, exercise becomes a time to celebrate life and discover the beauty that is within and around you. You look forward to it with excitement, enthusiasm and expectancy.

Different people are motivated by different desires. What makes one person feel passionate about exercise may leave another unaffected. One thing, though, is certain. The most potent desires are those that come from deep within our soul. These are the desires that arouse a heated passion within us and cause us to move forward with steadfast determination. Listed below are examples of both intrinsic and extrinsic desires or motivating factors that can be experienced from an active lifestyle. Read through them slowly and see which ones speak to you.

- Courage to confidently face life's challenges
- Strength to overcome any obstacle
- Vitality to breeze through the day with an invigorating aliveness
- Enthusiasm to attack all projects with passion
- An abundance of energy to easily accomplish what needs to be done
- A healthy self-esteem that brings confidence to all that I do
- Unbounded joy that fills my day with delightful experiences
- A deep peace that warms the soul
- Excellent health that causes my cells to dance in celebration
- A profound love that radiates from every cell of my being
- A self-confidence that allows me to step forward with excitement and anticipation
- A positive outlook that gives me encouragement
- A self-control that allows me to easily manage my thoughts
- A self-determination to accomplish anything I desire
- A greater awareness of the divinity that lies at the core of my being
- A greater realization/appreciation for the miracle of life
- The ability to easily focus on my heart's desire
- A passion for the possible, knowing limits exist only in my mind
- A genuine happiness that radiates from my heart at all times
- A greater ability to persist with focused determination
- Greater self-assurance to be proactive and move toward my most magnificent dreams

- Greater emotional freedom to release all hurts and negative thoughts

- Increased physical abilities to experience more of life with gusto

- Greater mental clarity to see clearly all the events of my life

- An unwavering hope for the future, knowing I live in a loving universe

- A greater ease of self-expression, allowing my true spirit to effortlessly unfold

- Greater creativity that brings a sense of adventure to all I undertake

- A greater acceptance of who I am, feeling gratitude and appreciation for the gift of life

- A deep compassion that fills my heart with love and warms my soul

- An inner beauty that puts a sparkle in my eyes and a smile on my face

The gifts you will receive from pursuing an active lifestyle with an intention that inspires are unlimited. Your entire life will expand to embrace more beauty and joy and you will feel a new zeal and enthusiasm fill your soul. Believe it. To assist you with imagining these possibilities, affirmations for each of the above benefits are listed in the appendix. Use these affirmations to help anchor the feelings in your heart, in your mind and in your body.

To review, making exercise a reality begins with knowing your starting point, developing a supportive environment, and discovering an intention that fills you with passion. When these are in place, you are now ready to construct a plan to implement your dreams.

4. Develop a Plan for the Possible

It has been said that failing to plan is planning to fail. I couldn't agree more. Most of us are creatures of habit, operating frequently on automatic pilot. If we customarily go home directly after work to prepare dinner and rush off to take care of other commitments, we will continue to do so unless we plan *ahead of time* to do something different. Without conscious planning, we often find ourselves slaves to our habits. So if we desire to make changes in our lifestyle and become more active, planning is an important and necessary step. The more time you spend methodically constructing a thorough plan, the greater your chances are of actually following through with it. But what exactly is involved in constructing such a meticulous plan?

The first thing is to approach the entire process with the attitude of excitement and anticipation. Instead of looking at planning as a routine task that will assist you in becoming more active, look upon it as an opportunity to deliberately design a new life, one that is filled with freedom, vitality, and joy. So planning is not only about scheduling exercise into your day, it's also about consciously choosing the direction you want your life to take and making the commitment to step in that direction with courage and confidence. Adopting this viewpoint makes it a lot easier—and a lot more fun—to make exercise a priority and squeeze it into an already busy day.

There are a number of factors that I have found helpful in designing a successful plan. These factors include: analyzing what you intend to do and when you intend to do it; making your exercise program as convenient as possible; and continuing to customize through journaling. Let's look at each of these in detail.

A. What and when.

The answers to what will you do and when will you do it are so interrelated that we will consider these two points together. Your favorite exercise may be swimming, but if you only have a total of 30 minutes that you can allot to your exercise program, swimming may not be possible. By the time you drive to a swimming pool and change into your swimsuit, you may find that you only have 60 seconds to actually exercise before you have to travel back home or to work. On the other hand, if swimming is not only your favorite exercise, but also the best and most comfortable exercise for you to do based on your current physical condition, then you may want to see how your schedule can be rearranged to accommodate this form of activity. Spend time looking at all the possibilities that come to mind. Sometimes the longer we ponder the possibilities, the more options we discover. Today we are virtually unlimited when it comes to choosing an exercise, especially with the huge DVD selections and the wide variety of community classes available. Explore all the alternatives available and choose the one that makes you feel good.

B. Make it convenient.

Convenience is one of the most important factors to consider in designing your exercise program. Making your exercise program convenient means making it easy to do and as fool-proof as possible, not leaving any doors open for excuses to walk in. If you have to drive through traffic to get to an exercise facility, or wake up an hour earlier to fit a workout in when you are definitely not a morning person, you may be setting yourself up for failure. But that doesn't mean it can't work. It means you need to brainstorm on ways to make it as easy as possible so that you stack the deck in your favor and follow through on your commitment.

Let's say that you happen to be a night owl, but morning is the only time you have available to exercise. There are a number of things you can do to make this plan work. To begin with, you might consider doing as much as you can the night before. This includes preparing all lunches, laying out both exercise and work clothes, and getting to bed earlier. Before going to bed, set the intention that you want to wake up fully rested and eager to start the day. This actually works! Another note: you don't have to be 100% awake to start exercising. During the summer, one of my greatest joys is watching the sunrise during my morning walk in the park. Sometimes, though, it seems to take almost 30 minutes of walking before my body actually feels awake. If you feel tired in the morning, begin exercising slowly and let your body dictate when to increase the intensity. By being gentle with yourself at this time of day, you may discover that morning becomes your favorite time to work out.

If morning workouts are out of the question and the evening is the only time you have available for exercising, there is still much you can do to make it more convenient. The challenges you may encounter with evening workouts include fatigue from the day, low blood sugar and lack of interest. So the first step is to address these challenges beforehand. You can combat fatigue and low blood sugar by always having healthy snacks available at work or in your car. Almonds and raisins, a health food bar or a protein drink work great as energy boosters. For the latter two, stay clear of any product that has high fructose corn syrup or evaporated cane juice in its list of ingredients. Both of these substances are disguised names for sugar. Additional energy boosters include apples, bananas or grapes with natural almond butter or a piece of organic cheese. Whether you snack on something at work or while driving home, the important thing is to make sure that when you arrive home, eating is not the first thing on your mind.

While driving home, keep your favorite CDs handy. These are the CDs that stimulate you into action, and rev up your engine. Even if you are carpooling, you can still listen to your personal selections on an MP3 player or iPod. Music is very powerful and can change your vibration in minutes. Use it to your advantage.

When you arrive home, you may still feel ambivalent about exercise so the trick is to act automatically and just do one step at a time. Immediately put on your exercise clothes—even if you still don't feel like exercising and can't imagine having the energy or desire to finish a workout. Tell yourself this is just the next step. You may not do the workout, but you can handle this next step. After you are dressed for exercise, begin by drinking some water. Often fatigue results from a state of mild dehydration, and drinking water can result in a quick energy boost. Next, do some simple stretches. Slow and easy, move your body, feeling the kinks that developed during the day loosening their hold. Breathe into the stretches in a leisurely manner. Remember, you still have not committed to doing the entire workout, but just taking this next step. Focus now on what you might gain from doing a gentle workout, keeping in mind some of the benefits previously mentioned. Will you feel more at peace, less stressful, more appreciative and grateful, or happy and energized? Now turn your attention to how you physically feel, and how the body is responding to the gentle stretching. If you still feel tired, tell yourself that you will just take one more step and do a little workout at an easy intensity. Then begin. Before you know it, a new surge of energy will fill your body and lift your spirits. With a little effort, you can finish your workout and feel the satisfaction of success.

The trick to the above scenario and taking one step at a time is to take these steps *automatically*. Just do it. Don't question it and let your mind debate it. Don't let your feelings get into it. Just take each step deliberately and automatically as if no other alternative existed. Then be prepared to pat yourself on the back after your workout.

Journaling your thoughts also helps, as described below in detail. Chances are you will feel refreshed, energized and good about yourself after your workout. Writing down these feelings will help you in the future when you feel the same reluctance to exercise. If you conquered your indifference to exercise once, you can do it again.

C. Customize through journaling.

When sailing from one destination to another, constant readjustment of the sails is necessary in order to stay on course. And so it is with any exercise program. What may seem like the perfect plan at the beginning of the week may turn out to be completely unworkable seven days later. Life is always changing, so your exercise plan needs to change along with it. One of the most effective tools that can help you customize your program to accommodate the changing circumstances of life is journaling.

The benefits of journaling are based on the *ink it, don't just think it* philosophy. There seems to be a certain power in the act of writing that brings to the conscious mind feelings and observations that would otherwise remain hidden. Through writing down your thoughts you can discover if your exercise program is too easy or too hard, if you are becoming bored or apathetic, if you need to refocus on your intention or if you need to strengthen your commitment. Journaling also helps bring all obstacles to the conscious level where you can then deal with them before they become potential problems. It lets you know what you need to change, empowering you to make the necessary adjustments.

Exactly what you journal is a personal preference but I have found that answering one or more of the following questions to be very helpful. A sample journal page can be found in the appendix.

> What did I do and how long did I do it?
> What were my feelings before, during and after my workout?
> What changes have I noticed (sleep patterns, stress levels, emotional, physical)?
> What worked?
> What didn't work?
> What needs to be changed?

By spending a few minutes answering these questions, you will discover what satisfies you and what doesn't satisfy you about your workout. You will find out what feeds your soul and what doesn't. You will learn what brings you pleasure and what drains your spirit. There is great wisdom in the *"Ink it, don't just think it"* philosophy. By taking a few minutes to jot down your thoughts and feelings, you will discover the valuable information you need to customize your exercise program and may also uncover some delightful surprises as well.

When talking with one of my clients some time ago about her exercise program, she responded that she was not getting any results. Upon questioning her, she did admit that she was sleeping much better, her stress levels were lower, her clothes were not as tight and she did have a bit more energy. But her focus was solely on the effect exercise was having on her weight. She had anticipated losing much more weight than what actually resulted from her efforts. This narrow focus kept her from realizing the many benefits that had indeed took place. Once she became aware of all that she had gained as a result of her exercise program, her enthusiasm for her workouts returned, and she went on to experience more success.

Journaling will not only unveil the many benefits that accompany the persistent pursuit of an exercise program, it will also highlight red flags that signal something needs to be changed. If you notice that boredom and apathy appear in your notations on a regular basis, adjustments are in order. You may need to reinforce your intention, change the activity you are doing or reassess when you are doing it. The more you tweak your program and customize it to bring you pleasure and satisfaction, the more you will increase your odds of success. The plan will work as long as you work the plan. Have fun with it and enjoy the results. For those who still aren't quite sure how to begin or would like more direction, a sample 30-day exercise plan can be found in the appendix.

5. Make it Fun

This is the only strategy that correlates closely with one of the steps (add pleasure and joy) for approaching exercise from a spiritual perspective. The reason it is repeated is because fun is absolutely necessary and a basic requirement for success. If exercise is merely another duty, responsibility or obligation, the chance of it being incorporated into your lifestyle is minimal. If it adds joy, laughter, happiness and pleasure, you won't have any problem making it a priority. So how do you make it fun if you've never enjoyed activity in the past? Simply do and add things that make you feel good. But first, adjust your perspective to allow for the possibility of fun.

Changing your perspective about exercise is important. Instead of looking upon it as exhausting work and a painful, uncomfortable experience, consider it a time to play, increase your inner strength and courage and raise your joy-quota. Become self-empowered. It can also be a time to release stress and anxiety. Seeing exercise from this perspective makes it more inviting, and opens your mind to look for ways to make it happen.

There are literally hundreds of different ways to exercise. You can walk, jog, bike, rollerblade, ski, dance, swim, follow an exercise video, attend a class, do yoga, t'ai chi, budokon, kickboxing, NIA, aerobics, circuit training, strength training, pilates, stretching, ball exercises, chair exercises, meridian exercises—the list is endless. If you haven't found enjoyment from exercise in the past, you may not have found the perfect form of exercise that soothes your soul. Do you like to work out alone or with others? Do you feel comfortable in an exercise class or do you prefer the privacy of your home? Do you need music or do you feel secure with your own thoughts? Remember, customize your program. You are totally in charge of what you do and how you progress. Begin with what makes you feel good.

If you are exercising at home, you can add fun to your workout by making the environment more enticing. A basement workout area can be spruced up with motivational posters, real or artificial plants and beautiful photographs of nature. Use your creativity. Sometimes, adding a name to the area and posting it on the wall helps. Instead of an exercise area, it could be a *Den of Discovery* or a *Palace of Possibilities*. We talked previously about the importance of the environment. This includes your exercise area. Spending the time to make it as pleasant as possible will make a huge difference in your attitude and the success of your program.

6. Do Something Daily.

During a t'ai chi class that I took several years ago, a visiting master shared the following story. There were two students who were both interested in the practice of t'ai chi. One student attended class regularly and practiced at home for an hour once a week. The other student also attended class regularly and practiced at home for five minutes every day. The master commented that the latter student who practiced for only five minutes, but on a daily basis, achieved the greater benefit for his effort. The master continued to explain that focusing on t'ai chi daily keeps the principles of t'ai chi in the forefront of the mind, allowing one to more fully embrace, and live from, these principles.

This same theory can be applied to exercise and self-empowerment. If some type of activity is done every day, exercise is not merely something that you do it also becomes a part of who you are. There are 288 five-minute segments in a 24-hour period. This step is asking you to use only one of these segments to send a message to the universe that you are committed to make a difference in your life. Before you become too alarmed with even the thought of daily activity, let me explain how easily this can be accomplished. Examples of daily activity include five minutes of stretching before or after your morning shower, or five minutes of deep breathing exercises when you need a break during the day. It could also mean performing one or two strength training exercises. In making the commitment to do something daily, the actual activity that you do may not matter as much as your commitment to do it. A daily commitment means you that you agree to make yourself a priority for five minutes every day. It instills in you a confidence that you *can* positively affect your health and encourages a proactive attitude that overflows into all areas of your life. It sends the message to the universe that no matter how busy life can be, you will always demand five minutes to spend on you and you alone. The regularity of doing some type of activity for five minutes every day is empowering, rewarding and relaxing, all at the same time. This is what a daily investment of five minutes can do. What a bargain!

7. Commit to Recommit

No matter how fool-proof you design a plan, chances are that at some point along the way a snag will occur. Your job changes, the washing machine breaks down, the kids get sick, your parents need help, or someone in the family is involved in an accident. Life can be unpredictable and demanding. Sometimes, no matter how strong your conviction is to follow through on your exercise program, implementation becomes impossible. You just can't seem to find any time at all.

When this happens, acknowledge it, accept it, and commit to recommit as soon as you can. It's important to remember to treat yourself with lovingkindness and compassion, and not identify with any negative, self-defeating thoughts. When you leave judgment out of the picture, it becomes much easier to restart your program. Just remember to commit to recommit.

When you strongly commit to something, including the idea to recommit, the universe rearranges itself to support you in every way possible. I discovered this principle many years ago while soaking in the breathtaking splendor of a magnificent sunset cruise in the Caribbean. My husband and I were on a small sailboat with the captain and his first mate. When the wine, cheese and crackers were being served I declined any of the refreshments stating that I was on a special diet. This was shortly after I started a macrobiotic diet and I was told to follow the diet for at least six months so that my body could rebuild itself. Not wanting the reoccurrence of any breathing problems, I made an unwavering commitment to meticulously follow the diet, even on our Caribbean vacation. To my absolute delight, the first mate was on the exact same diet and proceeded to produce a wonderful variety of the most delicious macrobiotic treats. He also shared with us the best restaurants to go to that served the type of food I could eat. The vacation turned out to be a glorious adventure and keeping my commitment became effortless.

According to a study with astronauts, it takes 30 days for the body to adopt to change. Hedge the odds in your favor, and make 60 days the critical period that you agree to consistently work your program. If you get interrupted, simply commit to recommit and start the 60 days over again. Remember you are a work in progress.

We are living in exciting times when so much is available to us as far as exercise options. It's also widely accepted now that exercise is an important part of a healthy lifestyle. No longer is physical activity reserved only for competitive athletes. Today it is an experience that is open to, and recommended for, all ages and all levels of physical abilities. Exercise is recognized as a universal human need. The question now is not if you are or are not exercising, but what type of exercise you are doing. Ride the wave of this burgeoning trend in self-responsibility and reap the benefits of an active lifestyle. Your spirit awaits you.

Seven Strategies for Success

Following is a quick summary of the strategies that will help you celebrate the joy of movement each and every day of your life. If you've gotten this far and have read the book to this point, you've already taken the first big step. All you have to do now is keep on going.

Success Strategy #1: Know your starting position. Take an honest look at your current state of health and fitness. Do this step without judgment, without being critical, without complaining—just observe.

Success Strategy #2: Adjust your environment. Whether it's your home, car, or workplace, create an environment that supports your efforts to lead a healthy, vibrant life. Release all that drains your energy and add whatever increases your vibration.

Success Strategy #3: Find an intention that inspires. Make the reason for embracing an active lifestyle one that ignites a passion deep within your soul. With a strong intention, remaining sedentary won't be an option. Reinforce your intention with affirmation cards at home, at work, in your car and in your wallet.

Success Strategy #4: Develop a Plan for the Possible. Design a plan that specifies what you will do and when you will do it. Ink it, don't just think it. Make it convenient. Continue to customize through journaling.

Success Strategy #5: Move with joy. Joy is the natural state of a free spirit. Whether it's through music, scenery or the activity itself, make sure joy enters every single workout.

Success Strategy #6: Do something daily. Make a declaration to the universe that you recognize your value as a divine being by spending at least 5 minutes each day on revitalizing your spirit. Whether it is deep breathing, stretching, balance exercises or a quick muscle toning routine, acknowledge your worth daily through movement.

Success Strategy #7: Commit to recommit. Life happens. Challenges appear, situations change, and the best devised plans fall by the wayside. As an old saying goes, when this happens, pick yourself up, dust yourself off and start all over again. Commit to recommit to your program for at least 60 days.

The Time is Now

There is one more story I'd like to share with you. This is the story of Clifford Young, an Australian potato farmer who lived on the outskirts of Melbourne. In 1983 at the age of 61 Cliff entered the inaugural Westfield Sydney to Melbourne race. This race covered a distance of 875 kilometers, or 542.5 miles, and was billed as being the world's toughest and longest ultra-marathon. Cliff believed in his heart he could go the distance. Others disagreed. In fact when he showed up at the start of the race in overalls and gumboots, most thought he was a publicity stunt. But Cliff was unaffected by what other people thought, and listened only to the voice that stirred within him.

Cliff's running style was as unconventional as his attire. Instead of a jog or run, his moves were more like a shuffle. As the race began the entire field of competitors left Cliff behind. He was in last place, yet he still continued to shuffle. To the astonishment of everyone, he shuffled passed all the competitors while they were sleeping, and five days, fifteen hours and four minutes later he shuffled his way to first place and won the race. In the years that followed that inaugural race, three other runners adopted what has come to be known as the "Young Shuffle" and each went on to win the race.

Cliff definitely marched to the beat of a different drummer. He followed his own inner guidance and enjoyed the liberty of being a free spirit. He gave away the $10,000 prize money for winning the race and continued this trend with all of his future winnings. He used his skill and notoriety to help others and became an advocate for local charities and non-profits, raising thousands of dollars throughout his racing career. Without a doubt, Cliff ran his own race and was lovingly known to those around him as an eccentric with a heart of gold.

Like Cliff, we all have a yearning in our soul that speaks to us when we quiet ourselves enough to listen. It is by listening to this yearning that we are given the opportunity to set our spirit free and experience a new way of being in this world. Wherever we are right now is the perfect place for us to begin. Through movement we have the power and the potential to change the course of our lives. By embracing our infinite creative potential we can step forward into a life filled with unlimited joy, radiant health, deep compassion and comforting peace. Physicist Dr. Richard Miller states that "As human beings we have extraordinary potentials we have hardly begun to study, much less understand." Use movement to help you explore this extraordinary potential and move forward with strength, courage and expectation to the life of your dreams. The time is now. Make your move and make it matter.

Movement is life
Exercise is movement.
So be alive,
And exercise!

APPENDIX A

▼

LIST OF ESSENTIAL OILS

Basil:	uplifting, refreshing
Bergamot:	uplifting, yet calming
Cedarwood:	relaxing, stress reducing
Eucalyptus:	invigorating, cleansing, tonifying, clearing
Frankincense:	calming, releasing fear, protecting
Geranium:	balancing mood swings, harmonizing
Juniper:	purifying, stimulating
Lavender:	calming, soothing, relaxing, balancing
Lemon:	uplifting, refreshing, energizing, cleansing
Lemongrass:	stimulating, cleansing, tonifying
Marjoram:	very relaxing, anxiety reducing, relieving
Patchouli:	inspiring, sensuous
Peppermint:	stimulating, cleansing, refreshing, invigorating, uplifting
Rose:	emotionally soothing
Rosemary:	stimulating, cleansing, invigorating
Sage:	cleansing, purifying
Sandalwood:	sensuous, soothing, helps release fear
Tea Tree:	disinfecting, stimulating

Thyme: stimulating, strengthening, activating

Ylang Ylang: sensuous, soothing

APPENDIX B

▼

AFFIRMATIONS

Acceptance
> *I completely and fully accept myself.*
> *I accept every aspect of my being, and know that Divine Source is always working through me.*
> *I accept all that life offers me with gratitude and appreciation.*

Appreciation
> *With gratitude and appreciation, I acknowledge the miracle of life.*
> *I honor all of life and appreciate its blessings.*
> *I appreciate the gift of all those who share my life.*

Compassion
> *I look upon others with love and compassion.*
> *I open my heart and compassionately respond to life's challenges.*
> *Compassion fills my entire being and I am at peace.*
> *I see only with love and compassion.*

Courage
> *I confidently step forward with courage.*
> *I courageously move forward in my life with, knowing I have the full support of the universe.*
> *I courageously embrace all the challenges in my life.*

Creativity
> *I enjoy creating and have a constant supply of fresh ideas.*

I am a creative spirit.
I bring creativity to all my endeavors.
I easily create the environment I desire.

Discipline

I easily and effortlessly follow through with my goals.
My character is strong and steadfast.
I am able to efficiently accomplish what I desire.

Energy

I have an abundance of energy to do all I need to do.
I easily go through my day with unlimited energy.
I feel energized as I move through my day.

Emotional freedom

I release all thoughts that are not for my highest good.
I let go of all fear and anger.
I am free from negative emotions, and release past hurts.
I connect to my inner wisdom and allow divine understanding to guide my thoughts.
I am guided by my inner wisdom in all my thoughts and actions.

Enthusiasm

My body sizzles with enthusiasm.
I eagerly anticipate each new day, filled with zeal and enthusiasm.
I am energized by my thoughts, and feel a wave of enthusiasm flood my body.

Focus/concentration

I easily focus on the task at hand.
My ability to concentrate is increasing daily.
I am clear and focused in the pursuit of my goals.

Happiness

Happiness and joy are my natural state and I experience them daily.
All the cells of my body tingle with happiness.
I am surrounded by happiness and rejoice in it.
I bring happiness to all my endeavors.

Health

I celebrate my healthy and strong body.

As my health improves, I see divine perfection reflected in my body.
Each day I give thanks for my healthy body.
My body is getting better and better, every day in every way.

Hope

I overcome my challenges with hope and courage.
My hope sustains me through tough times.
My hope for the future is strong and unwavering.

Inner beauty

The radiance of my soul shines brightly.
I allow my inner beauty to shine forth, providing a guiding light for others.
My essence is love, and it floods my entire being.

Joy

I celebrate life with an abundance of joy and enthusiasm.
I embrace life with unbridled joy.
I am filled with joy and feel it deep within my being.
I am now living in the presence of joy and know joy is my natural state.
I feel joy flowing through every cell of my being.
I let the song of joy fill my heart and celebrate its presence.

Love

I am a spark of the divine, and love is my true essence.
I am worthy of all the love in the universe.
I open my heart and easily embrace love.
It is safe for me to give and receive love.
I am surrounded by love and see love in all that surrounds me.
I now radiate with deep feelings of love.

Mental clarity

My mind is sharp and clear.
I perceive all that is around me with clarity.
I release all mental chatter, leaving my mind clear and peaceful.

Passion

I embrace life with passion and enthusiasm.
I am filled with passion and an excitement for life.
I passionately pursue my dreams and see them becoming my reality.

Peace

> *I trust the process of life and am at peace.*
> *I release all my fears and feel a comforting peace fill my being.*
> *I am at peace and all is well.*
> *I choose to live in perfect peace, with honor and integrity.*
> *Peace, harmony and beauty forever live within me.*

Persistence

> *I will persist until I succeed.*
> *I persistently pursue my deepest desires.*
> *I follow through with persistence and determination.*

Physical health

> *My body is getting stronger, everyday in everyway.*
> *I am flexible and bend with grace and ease.*
> *My heart is strong and provides me with an abundance of energy.*
> *I can physically accomplish anything I set my mind to do.*

Positive outlook

> *I look for the positive in all that life brings me.*
> *I am positive and optimistic about life.*
> *I live in a universe that always supports me.*

Satisfaction

> *I feel good about my life.*
> *I always do my best and am satisfied with the results.*
> *I am content with my life and know that everything is in divine order.*
> *I accept my present life while I work to improve it.*

Self-confidence

> *With confidence, I easily move forward in life.*
> *I believe in me.*
> *I am confident that I can accomplish all that is mine to do.*

Self-control

> *I am the master of all my thoughts and actions.*
> *I easily and effortlessly manage my life.*
> *I am in control of all my actions and always act in my highest good.*

Self-determination

With unwavering conviction, I move forward in my life.
I proceed with all tasks with conviction and deep resolve.
I accomplish my goals with steadfast determination.

Self-esteem

I love and approve of myself everyday in every way.
I am a divine being.
I am worthy of all the good in the universe.

Self-expression

I allow my unique spirit to fully express itself.
I am an individual expression of the divine, and let my radiance glow.
I comfortably let my true spirit unfold.

Spiritual connection

I am a spiritual being having a human experience.
I am a spark of the Divine, and radiate peace and love.
Divine love is my source, and I easily connect with that Source daily.

Strength

I am stronger than any challenge.
With strength, I will persist until I succeed.
I easily move forward with strength and determination.
The strength of the entire universe resides within me.

Vitality

My body is alive with a new and vibrant energy.
I celebrate the abundance of vitality that fills my body.
I am filled with excitement and vitality as I go through my day.

APPENDIX C

▼

30-DAY FLIGHT PLAN

Preparation

Theme: Anticipation
Affirmation: *I eagerly prepare for new adventures in my life.*

Spend at least one week, but no longer than one month, making the necessary preparations for whatever you require to insure your success. Some of the things you might address include: clearing clutter, developing affirmations and purchasing clothing or equipment such as shoes, exercise videos, or CDs. Begin this program on a Monday. When preparation is complete, proceed to Week 1.

Week 1

Theme: Conscious creating
Affirmation: *I embrace the present moment with love and through my thoughts create a radiant and beautiful life.*
Lifestyle change: Soak in an Epsom salt bath one day this week. Release into the bath water all that is not for your highest good.

Monday:	Daily dose—breathing exercises, 5 minutes Walk, 20 minutes*
Tuesday:	Daily dose—breathing exercises, 5 minutes

*Whenever walking is stated you may substitute any other aerobic activity.

Wednesday:	Daily dose—breathing exercises, 5 minutes Walk, 20 minutes
Thursday:	Daily dose—breathing exercises, 5 minutes
Friday:	Daily dose—breathing exercises, 5 minutes Walk, 20 minutes
Saturday:	Daily dose—breathing exercises, 5 minutes
Sunday:	Daily dose—breathing exercises, 5 minutes Evaluate program and progress. Repeat week 1 or move to week 2

Week 2

Theme: Awareness
Affirmation: *I am uplifted by the presence of the divine in every cell of my body. I am a divine masterpiece and celebrate my perfection.*
Lifestyle change: Drink four or more glasses of water per day with a slice of lemon in at least one of the glasses of water.

Monday:	Daily dose—breathing exercises, 5 minutes Walk, 20 minutes
Tuesday:	Daily does—strength exercises for arms, 5 minutes
Wednesday:	Daily dose—breathing exercises, 5 minutes Walk, 30 minutes
Thursday:	Daily dose—strength exercises for legs, 5 minutes
Friday:	Daily dose—breathing exercises, 5 minutes Walk, 20 minutes
Saturday:	Daily dose—breathing exercises, 5 minutes
Sunday:	Daily dose—breathing exercises, 5 minutes Evaluate program and progress. Repeat week 2 or move to week 3.

Week 3

Theme: Courage and strength
Affirmation: *I step forward with strength and courage fully committed to my path of love and light.*

Lifestyle change: Eliminate TV, radio and newspapers for the entire week. Replace them with positive movies and videos, CDs, books and magazines.

Monday:	Daily dose—strength exercises for back, 5 minutes Walk, 25 minutes
Tuesday:	Daily dose—breathing exercises, 5 minutes
Wednesday:	Daily dose—strength exercises for chest, 5 minutes Walk, 35 minutes
Thursday:	Daily dose—breathing exercises, 5 minutes
Friday:	Daily dose—strength exercises for shoulders, 5 minutes Walk, 25 minutes
Saturday:	Daily dose—stretching exercises, 5 minutes
Sunday:	Daily dose—stretching exercises, 5 minutes Evaluate program and progress. Repeat week 3 or move to week 4.

Week 4

Theme: Connectedness
Affirmation: *I am centered in unshakable peace and feel a connection to all of life that calms my soul.*
Lifestyle change: Smile at everyone you encounter during the entire week.

Monday:	Daily dose—breathing exercises, 5 minutes Walk, 30 minutes
Tuesday:	Daily dose—stretching exercises, 5 minutes
Wednesday:	Daily dose—breathing exercises, 5 minutes Walk, 40 minutes
Thursday:	Daily dose—stretching exercises, 5 minutes
Friday:	Daily dose—breathing exercises, 5 minutes Walk, 30 minutes
Saturday:	Daily dose—stretching exercises, 5 minutes
Sunday:	Daily dose—stretching exercises, 5 minutes Evaluate program and progress. Repeat week 4 or move to week 5

Week 5

Theme: Celebration

Affirmation: *I rejoice in the miracle of life and celebrate the beauty and excitement of my transformation.*

Lifestyle change: Eat and drink only home-cooked food and beverages.

Monday:	Daily dose—breathing exercises, 5 minutes Walk, 40 minutes
Tuesday:	Daily dose—breathing exercises, 5 minutes Walk 40 minutes Evaluate 30 day program. Make appropriate adjustments to accommodate your comfort level and goals.

Appendix D

▼

Walking Program—Minutes

	Day 1	Day 2	Day 3	Day 4	Total Time
Week 1	20	25	15	30	90
Week 2	22	27	17	32	98
Week 3	25	30	20	35	110
Week 4	27	32	22	37	118
Week 5	30	35	25	40	130

Keep in Mind:

- Always warm up by starting slowly and gradually increasing your speed.

- Always cool down by gradually decreasing your speed and stretching.

- Never skip more than two days in a row or walk more than 3 days in a row.

- Day 3 is a great day to pick up your pace since the walking time is the shortest.

- Day 4 is a great day to decrease your pace since the walking time is the longest.

Appendix E

▼

Taking Flight Journal Page

Day/Date: _____
List the type of activity performed and the length of the workout.

_____

_____

Briefly describe your feelings before, during and after your workout?

_____

_____

_____

What changes have I noticed (sleep patterns, stress levels, emotional, physical)?

_____

_____

_____

What worked?

_____

_____

_____

_____

What didn't work?

_____

_____

_____

_____

_____

What needs to be changed?

_____

_____

_____

If it's going to be, it's up to me!

_____

About the Author

"Darlene Danko Sowa is an exercise physiologist and certified healing touch practitioner whose passion has been to help people explore their divine potential through movement. In 1985 she co-founded Professional Fitness Systems, a company that provided a wide range of wellness services. For the next 18 years she spearheaded dozens of wellness programs in both the corporate and community setting. She was appointed to the Michigan Governor's Council on Physical Fitness and Sports and served two terms working to promote a healthy and active community. Her healing journey led her to an interest in energy medicine and certification as a healing touch practitioner.

Darlene currently operates a private practice in Michigan where she happily resides with her husband, Tom, and their golden retriever, Gilda. She continues to conduct workshops and speak on *Exercising with Spirit* and can be reached at darstar1@sbcglobal.net.

978-0-595-47527-8
0-595-47527-2

Printed in the United States
201983BV00002B/1-51/A